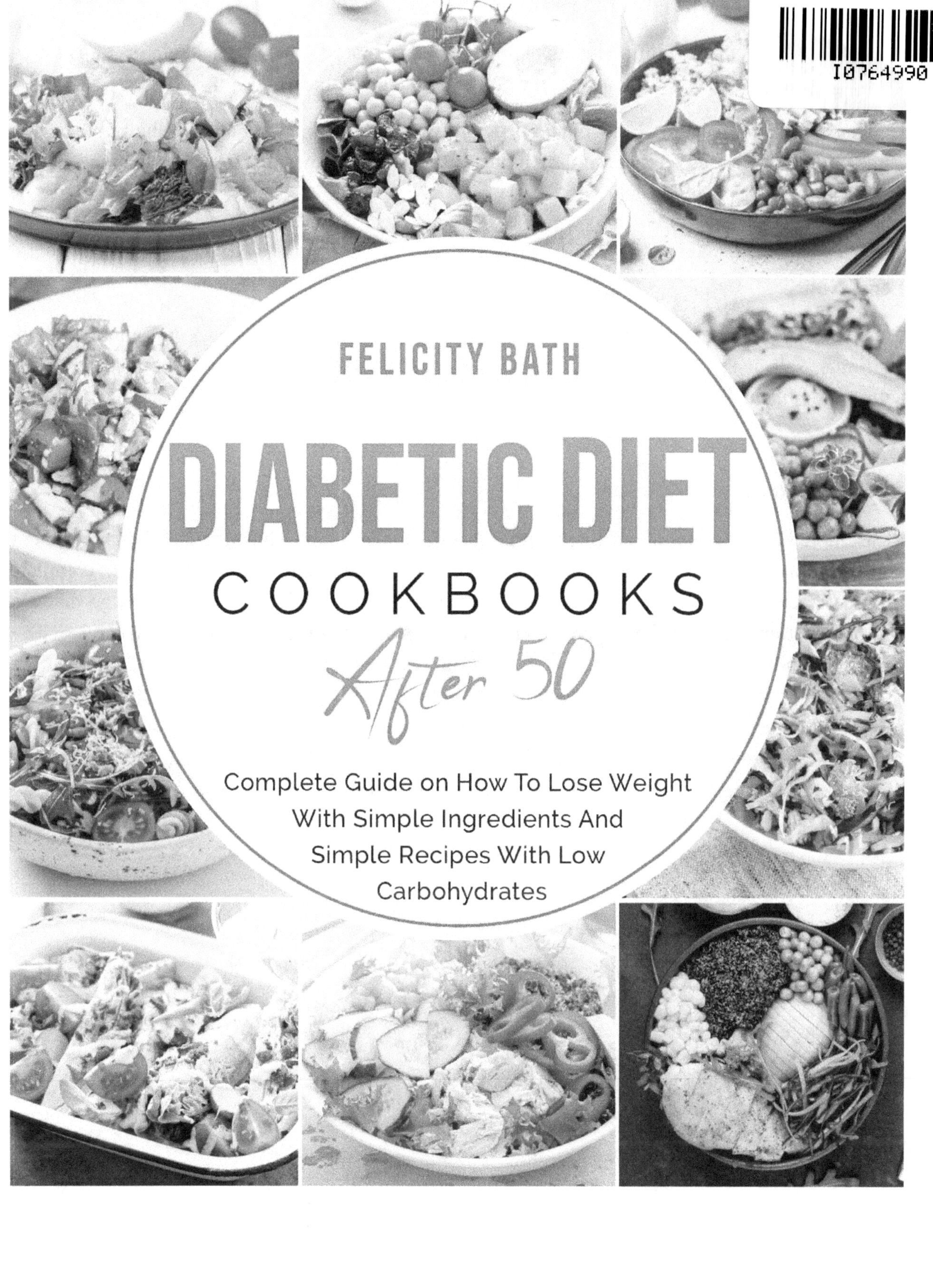

FELICITY BATH
DIABETIC DIET
COOKBOOKS
After 50
Complete Guide on How To Lose Weight
With Simple Ingredients And
Simple Recipes With Low
Carbohydrates

TABLE OF CONTENTS

DIABETICS DIET COOKBOOKS AFTER 50

COMPLETE GUIDE ON HOW TO LOSE WEIGHT WITH INGREDIENT AND SIMPLE RECIPE WITH LOW CARBOHYDRATE

INTRODUCTION ON HEALTHY EATING

Eating well is fundamental to good health and well-being. Healthy eating helps us to maintain a healthy weight. It reduces our risk of diabetes, high blood pressure, high cholesterol, and the risk of developing cardiovascular disease and some cancers.

WHY IS EATING WELL IMPORTANT?

Healthy eating has many other benefits. When we eat well, we sleep better, have more energy, and better concentration – and this all adds up to healthier, happier lives! Healthy eating should be an enjoyable social experience. When children and young people eat and drink well, they get all the essential nutrients they need to develop and develop a good relationship with food and other social skills.

What is healthy eating?

Healthy eating isn't about cutting out foods – it's about eating a wide variety of foods in the right amounts to give your body what it needs. There are no available foods you must eat or menus you need to follow to eat healthily. You just need to make sure you get the right balance of different foods. Healthy eating for children and young people should always include a range of exciting and tasty food that can make up a healthy, varied, and balanced diet, rather than denying them certain foods and drinks. Although all foods can be included in a healthy diet, this will not be true for special/medical diets.

What are the benefits of eating healthy?

A healthful diet includes various fruits and vegetables of many colors, whole grains and starches, good fats, and lean proteins. Eating healthfully also means avoiding foods with high amounts of added salt and sugar.

We look at the top 10 benefits of a healthful diet, as well as the evidence behind them.

1. Weight loss

Losing weight can help to reduce the risk of chronic conditions. If a person is overweight or obese, they have a higher risk of developing several conditions, including:

- Heart Disease
- Non-Insulin-Dependent Diabetes Mellitus
- Poor Bone Density
- Some Cancers

Whole vegetables and fruits are lower in calories than most processed foods. A person looking to lose weight should reduce their calorie intake to no more than what they require each day.

Maintaining a healthful diet free from processed foods can help a person stay within their daily limit without counting calories. Fiber is one element of a healthful diet that is particularly important for managing weight. Plant-based foods contain plenty of dietary FiberFiber, regulating hunger by making people feel fuller for longer.

In 2018, researchers found that a diet rich in FiberFiber and lean proteins resulted in weight loss without the need for counting calories.

2. Reduced cancer risk

An unhealthful diet can lead to obesity, which may increase a person's risk of developing cancer. Weighing within a healthful range may reduce this risk.

In 2014, the American Society of Clinical Oncology reported that obesity contributed to a worse outlook for people with cancer.

However, diets rich in fruits and vegetables may help to protect against cancer.

In a separate study from 2014, researchers found that a diet rich in fruits reduced the risk of cancers of the upper gastrointestinal tract. They also found that a diet rich in vegetables, fruits, and FiberFiber lowered the risk of colorectal cancer and that a diet rich in FiberFiber reduced the risk of liver cancer.

Many phytochemicals found in fruits, vegetables, nuts, and legumes act as antioxidants, which protect cells from damage that can cause cancer. Some of these antioxidants include beta-carotene, lycopene, and vitamins A, C, and E.

Trials in humans have been inconclusive, but results of laboratory and animal studies have linked certain antioxidants to a reduced incidence of free radical damage associated with cancer.

3. Diabetes management

Eating a healthful diet can help a person with diabetes to:

- Lose Weight, If Required
- Manage Blood Glucose Levels
- Keep Blood Pressure And Cholesterol Within Target Ranges Prevent Or Delay Complications Of Diabetes

It is essential for people with diabetes to limit their intake of foods with added sugar and salt. It is also best to avoid fried foods high in saturated and trans fats.

4. Heart health and stroke prevention

According to figures published in 2017, as many as 92.1 million people in the U.S. have at least one type of cardiovascular disease. These conditions primarily involve the heart or blood vessels.

According to the Heart and Stroke Foundation of Canada, up to 80 percent of premature heart disease and stroke cases can be prevented by making lifestyle changes, such as increasing levels of physical activity and eating healthfully.

There is some evidence that vitamin E may prevent blood clots, which can lead to heart attacks. The following foods contain high levels of vitamin E:

- Almonds
- Peanuts
- Hazelnuts
- Sunflower Seeds
- Green Vegetables

The medical community has long recognized the link between trans fats and heart-related illnesses, such as coronary heart disease.

If a person eliminates trans fats from the diet, this will reduce their low-density lipoprotein cholesterol levels. This type of cholesterol causes plaque to collect within the arteries, increasing heart attack, and stroke risk.

Reducing blood pressure can also be essential for heart health, and limiting salt intake to 1,500 milligrams a day can help.

Salt is added to many processed and fast foods, and a person hoping to lower their blood pressure should avoid these.

5. The health of the next generation

Children learn most health-related behaviors from the adults around them, and parents who model healthful eating and exercise habits tend to pass these on.

Eating at home may also help. In 2018, researchers found that children who regularly had meals with their families ate more vegetables and fewer sugary foods than their peers who ate at home less frequently.

Also, children who participate in gardening and cooking at home may be more likely to make healthful dietary and lifestyle choices.

6. Strong bones and teeth

A diet with adequate calcium and magnesium is necessary for strong bones and teeth. Keeping the bones healthy is vital in preventing osteoporosis and osteoarthritis later in life.

The following foods are rich in calcium:

- Low-Fat Dairy Products
- Broccoli
- Cauliflower
- Cabbage
- Canned Fish With Bones
- Tofu
- Legumes

Also, many bowls of cereal and plant-based milk are fortified with calcium.

Magnesium is abundant in many foods, and the best sources are leafy green vegetables, nuts, seeds, and whole grains.

7. Better mood

Emerging evidence suggests a close relationship between diet and mood.

In 2016, researchers found that a diet with a high glycemic load may increase depression and fatigue symptoms.

A diet with a high glycemic load includes many refined carbohydrates, such as those found in soft drinks, cakes, white bread, and biscuits. Vegetables, whole fruit, and whole grains have a lower glycemic load.

While a healthful diet may improve overall mood, people with depression need to seek medical care.

8. Improved memory

A healthful diet may help prevent dementia and cognitive decline.

A study from 2015 identified nutrients and foods that protect against these adverse effects. They found the following to be beneficial:

- Vitamin D, C, And E
- Omega-3 Fatty Acids
- Flavonoids And Polyphenols
- Fish

Among other diets, the Mediterranean diet incorporates many of these nutrients.

9. Improved gut health

The colon is full of naturally occurring bacteria, which play essential roles in metabolism and digestion.

Certain strains of bacteria also produce vitamins K and B, which benefit the colon. These strains also help to fight harmful bacteria and viruses.

A diet low in FiberFiber and high in sugar and fat alters the gut microbiome, increasing inflammation in the area.

However, a diet rich in vegetables, fruits, legumes, and whole grains provides a combination of prebiotics and probiotics that help good bacteria to thrive in the colon.

Fermented foods, such as Yogurt, kimchi, sauerkraut, miso, and kefir, are rich in probiotics. Fiber is an easily accessible prebiotic, and it is abundant in legumes, grains, fruits, and vegetables.

Fiber also promotes regular bowel movements, which can help to prevent bowel cancer and diverticulitis.

10. Getting a good night's sleep

A variety of factors, including sleep apnea, can disrupt sleep patterns.

Sleep apnea occurs when the airways are repeatedly blocked during sleep. Risk factors include obesity, drinking alcohol, and eating an unhealthy diet.

Reducing alcohol and caffeine consumption can help to ensure restful sleep, whether or not a person has sleep apnea.

Quick tips for a healthful diet

There are plenty of small, positive ways to improve the diet, including:

- Swapping Soft Drinks For Water And Herbal Tea
- Eating No Meat For At Least One Day A Week
- Ensuring That Produce Makes Up About 50 Percent Of Each Meal
- Swapping Cow's Milk For Plant-Based Milk
- Eating Whole Fruits Instead Of Drinking Juices, Which Contain Less Fiberfiber And Often Include Added Sugar
- Avoiding Processed Meats, Which Are High In Salt And May Increase The Risk Of Colon Cancer
- Eating More Lean Protcin, Which Can Be Found In Eggs, Tofu, Fish, And Nuts

A person may also benefit from taking a cooking class and learning how to incorporate more vegetables into meals. A doctor or dietitian can also provide tips on eating a more healthful diet.

A GUIDE TO HEALTHY LOW CARB EATING WITH DIABETES

Diabetes is a chronic disease that affects many people across the globe. Currently, more than 400 million people have diabetes worldwide.

Although diabetes is a complicated disease, maintaining adequate blood sugar levels can significantly reduce the risk of complications.

One of the ways to achieve better blood sugar levels is to follow a low carb diet. This article provides a detailed overview of deficient carb diets for managing diabetes. With diabetes, the body can't effectively process carbohydrates.

Usually, when you eat carbs, they're broken down into small glucose units, which end up as blood sugar. When blood sugar levels go up, the pancreas responds by producing the hormone insulin. This hormone allows blood sugar to enter cells.

What IS DIABETES, AND WHAT ROLE DOES FOOD PLAY?

With diabetes, the body can't effectively process carbohydrates. Usually, when you eat carbs, they're broken down into small glucose units, which end up as blood sugar.

When blood sugar levels go up, the pancreas responds by producing the hormone insulin. This hormone allows blood sugar to enter cells. In people without diabetes, blood sugar levels remain within a narrow range throughout the day. For those who have diabetes, however, this system doesn't work in the same way. This is a big problem because having both too high and too low blood sugar levels can cause severe harm.

There are several types of diabetes, but the two most common ones are type 1 and type 2 diabetes. Both of these conditions can occur at any age.

In type 1 diabetes, an autoimmune process destroys the insulin-producing beta cells in the pancreas. People with diabetes take insulin several times a day to ensure that glucose gets into the cells and stays healthy in the bloodstream.

In type 2 diabetes, the beta cells at first produce enough insulin, but the body's cells are resistant to its action, so blood sugar remains high. To compensate, the pancreas produces more insulin, attempting to bring blood sugar down.

Over time, the beta cells lose their ability to produce enough insulin. Of the three macronutrients — protein, carbs, and fat — carbs significantly impact blood sugar management. This is because the body breaks them down into glucose. Therefore, people with diabetes may need to take large doses of insulin, medication, or both when they eat many carbohydrates.

Can Deficient Carb Diets Help Manage Diabetes?

Many studies support low carb diets for the treatment of diabetes. In fact, before discovering insulin in 1921, deficient carb diets were considered standard treatment for people with diabetes.

What's more, low carb diets seem to work well in the long term when people stick to them. In one study, people with type 2 diabetes ate a low carb diet for six months. Their diabetes remained well managed more than three years later if they stuck to the diet.

Similarly, when people with type 1 diabetes followed a carb-restricted diet, those who followed the diet saw a significant improvement in blood sugar levels over four years.

A LOW-CARB DIET AND MEALPLAN

Eating a low-carb diet means cutting down on the number of carbohydrates (carbs) you eat to less than 130g a day. But low-carb eating shouldn't be no-carb eating.

Some carbohydrate foods contain essential vitamins, minerals, and FiberFiber, which form an essential part of a healthy diet.

Here we'll explain what we mean by low-carb, the benefits of low-carb eating when you have diabetes, and share a low-carb meal plan to help you get started if this is the diet for you. We'll also explain how to get support to manage any potential risks, especially if you manage your diabetes with medications that put you at risk of hypos.

If you or someone you know is self-isolating, find out how to eat healthily while staying at home.

What's A Low-Carb Diet?

But how low is low-carb? There are different types of low-carb diets. Generally, low-carb eating reduces the total amount of carbs you consume in a day to less than 130g.

To put this into context, a medium-sized slice of bread is about 15 to 20g of carbs, which is about the same as a regular apple. On the other hand, a large jacket potato could have as much as 90g of carbs, as does one liter of orange juice.

A low-carb diet isn't for everyone. The most substantial evidence we have to show the benefits of low-carb diets is in adults with obesity and those with type 2 diabetes who need to lose weight. If you decide to follow a low-carb diet, it's essential to know all the potential benefits and manage any potential risks.

Low-Carb Meal Plan

There's no one-size-fits-all for choosing a meal plan. Before you begin any healthy eating program, please read our guide on choosing your meal plan to ensure you follow the plan that's right for you.

Our low-carb meal plan aims to help you maintain a healthy balance while reducing the number of carbs you eat. Varying amounts of carbohydrates are shown each day to help you choose which works best for you. It's nutritionally balanced, we've counted the calories for you, and it contains at least five portions of fruit and veg per day.

Low-Carb Diet

Monday's low-carb meal plan

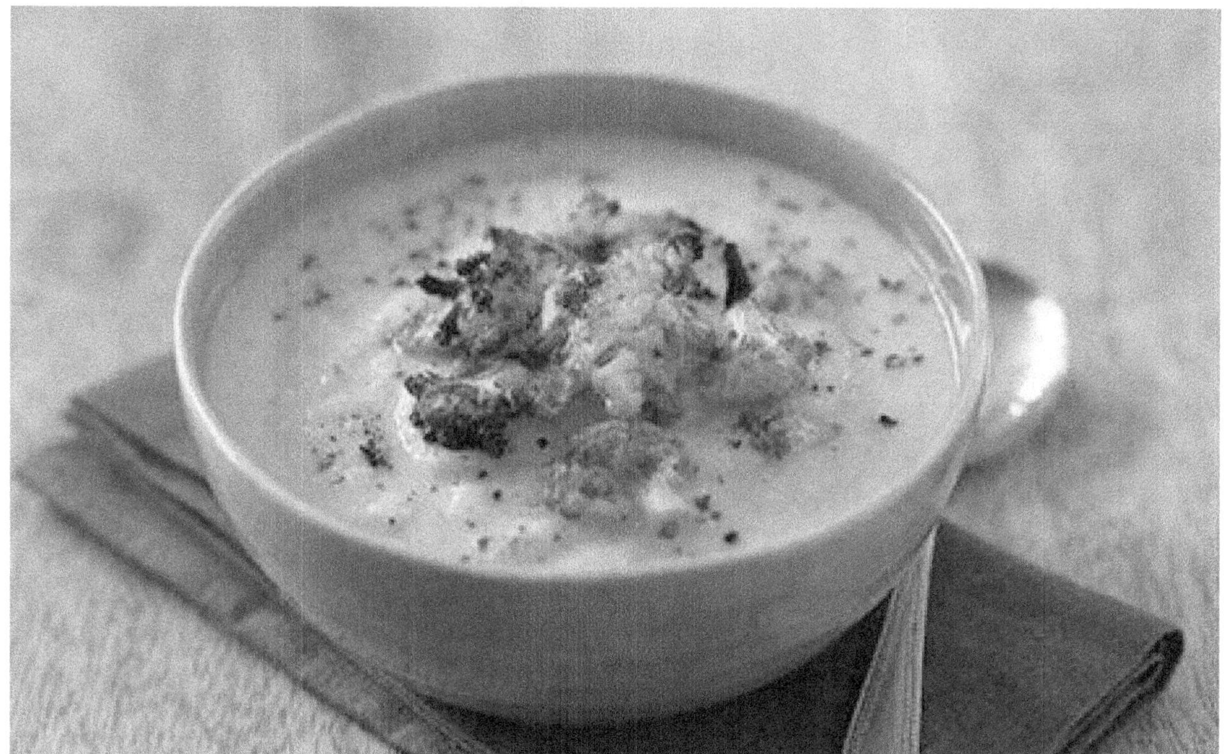

Breakfast: Wholemeal toast with scrambled eggs

Lunch: Cauliflower and leek soup

Dinner: Lower-fat Cauliflower and broccoli cheese with a medium grilled salmon fillet

Pudding: Greek Yogurt with raspberries

Choose from snacks, including fruit, nuts, and rye crackers with avocado.

Tuesday's low-carb meal plan

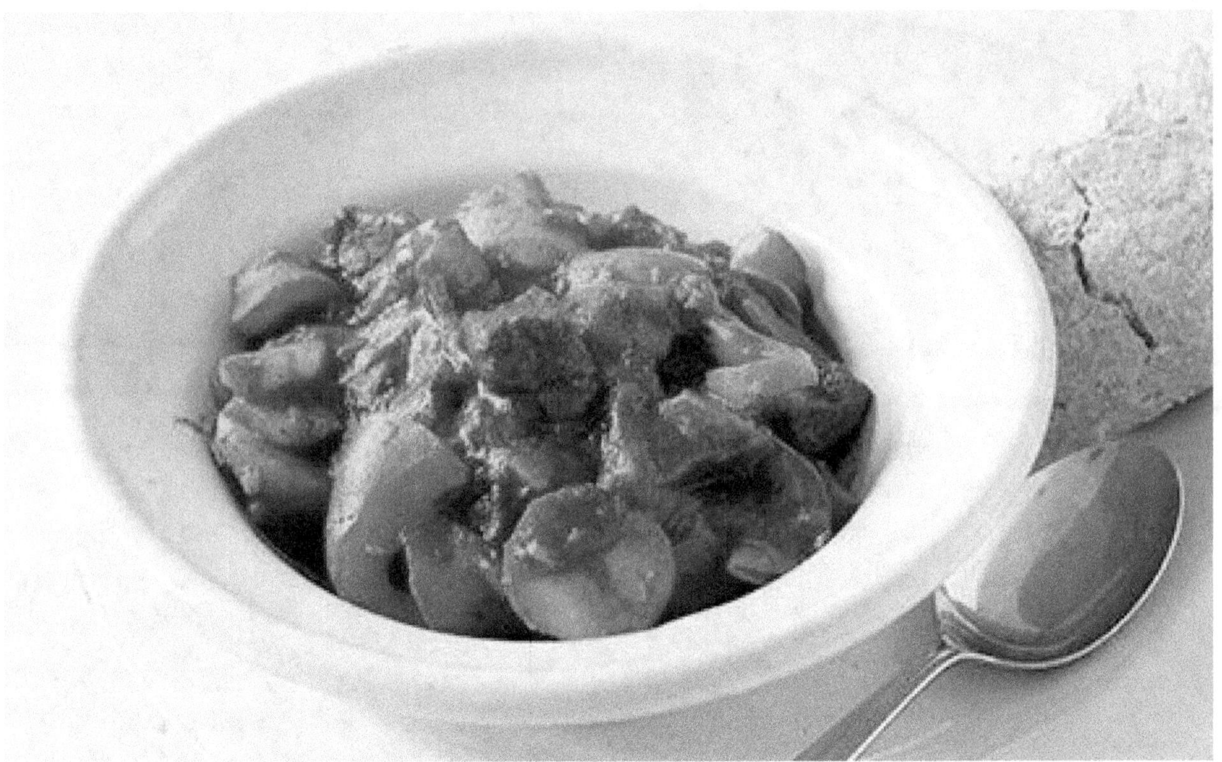

Breakfast: Greek Yogurt with raspberries and pumpkin seeds

Lunch: Chickpea and tuna salad and strawberries

Dinner: Beef goulash

Pudding: Rhubarb fool

Choose from snacks, including granary bread with peanut butter, avocado, Greek Yogurt, crudites, and nuts.

Wednesday's low-carb meal plan

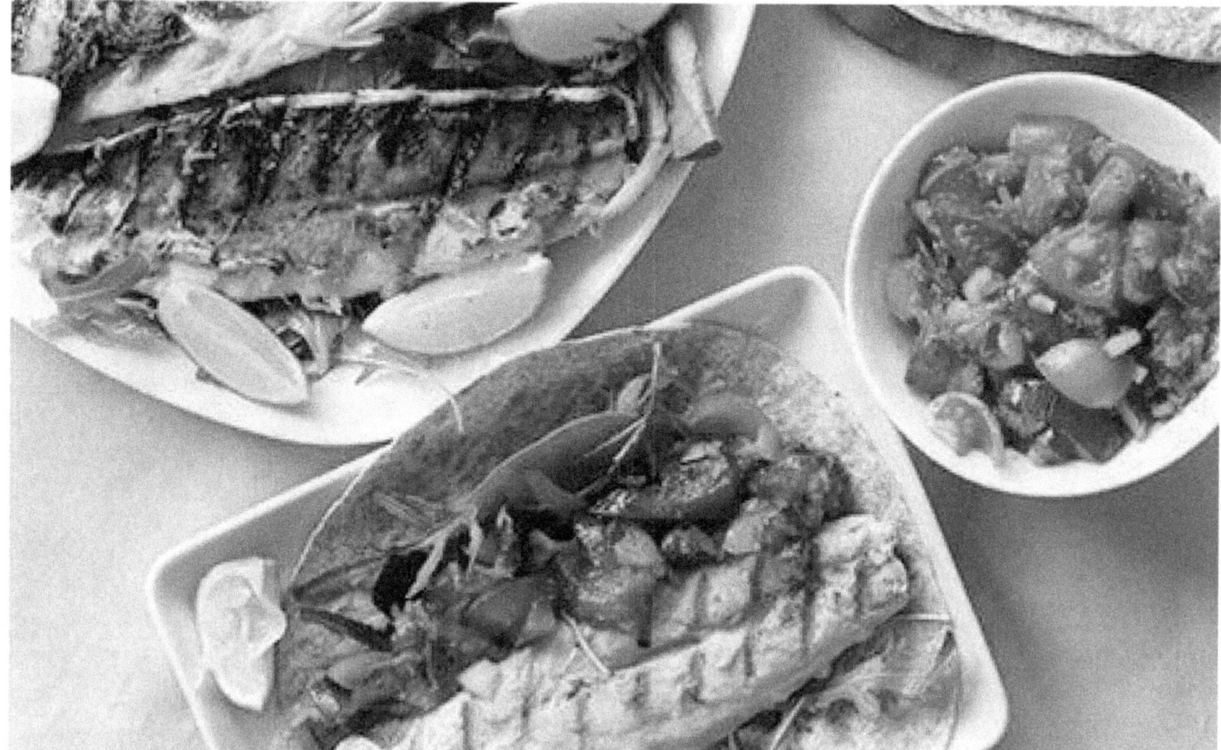

Breakfast: Porridge with almonds, blueberries, and pumpkin seeds

Lunch: Mackerel salsa wrap

Dinner: Chicken casserole with Broccoli

Pudding: Greek Yogurt with strawberries and blueberries

Choose from snacks, including nuts, wholemeal rice cakes with peanut butter, and crudites with guacamole.

Thursday's low-carb meal plan

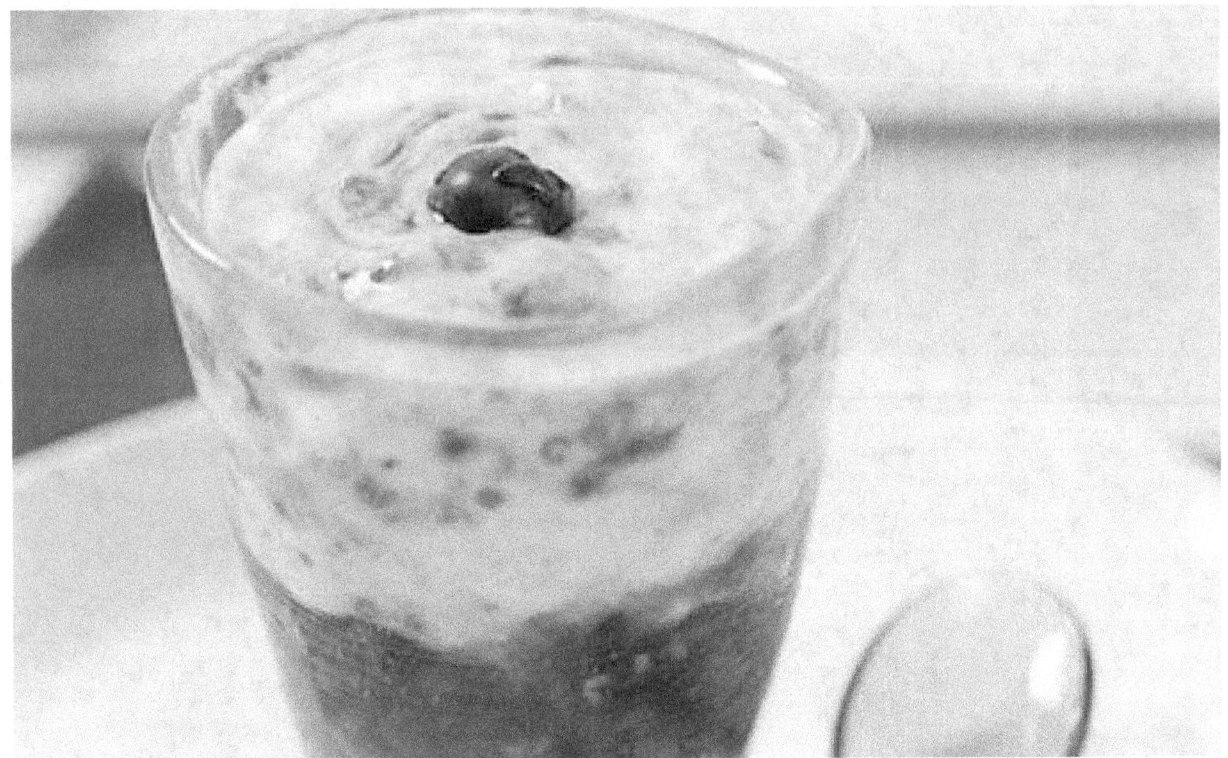

Breakfast: Mushroom omelet with mushrooms and grilled tomato

Lunch: Creamy chicken and mushroom soup and Greek Yogurt with raspberries

Dinner: Beefburger with a green salad

Pudding: Summer berry posset

Choose from snacks, including oatcakes with light cream cheese, nuts, and avocado.

Friday's low-carb meal plan

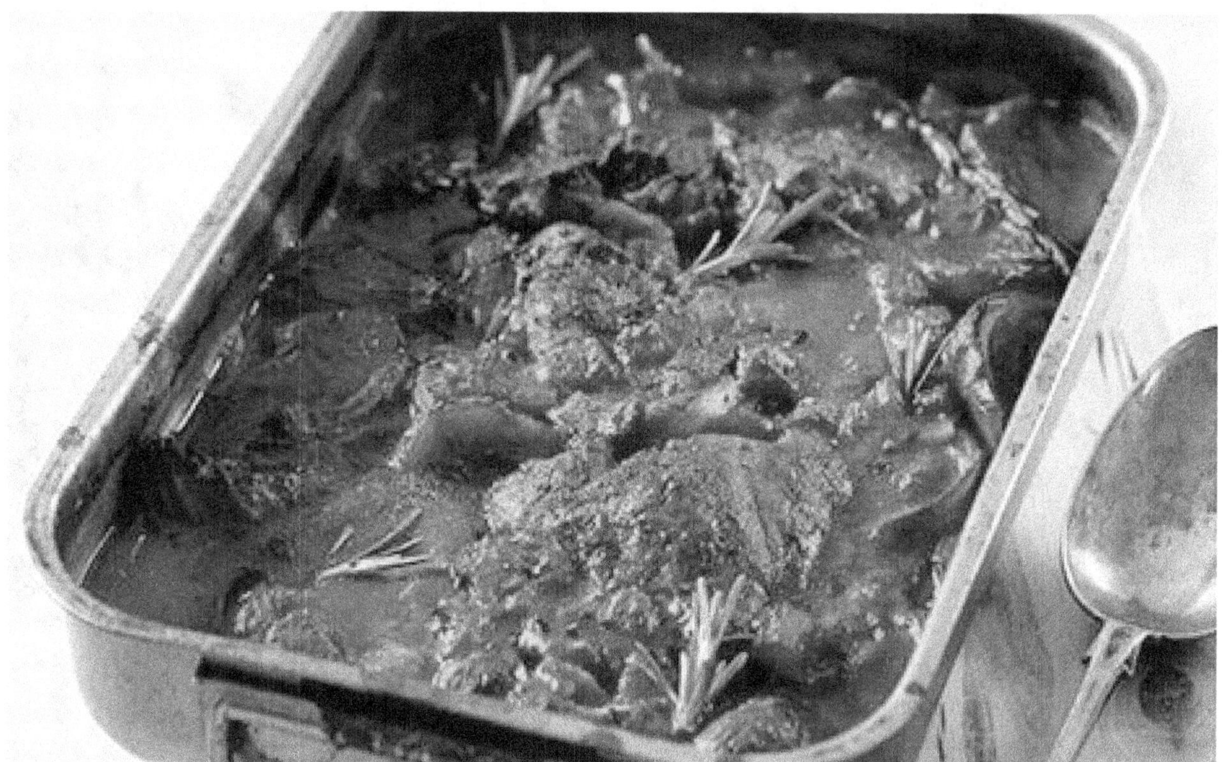

Breakfast: Scrambled egg on granary toast with mushrooms

Lunch: Beef and barley soup and Greek Yogurt

Dinner: Italian-style braised lamb steaks with brown rice and Broccoli

Pudding: Microwave mug: Chocolate, banana, and almond cup with half-fat creme fraiche

Choose from snacks, including nuts, cheese, and guacamole with crudites.

Saturday's low-carb meal plan

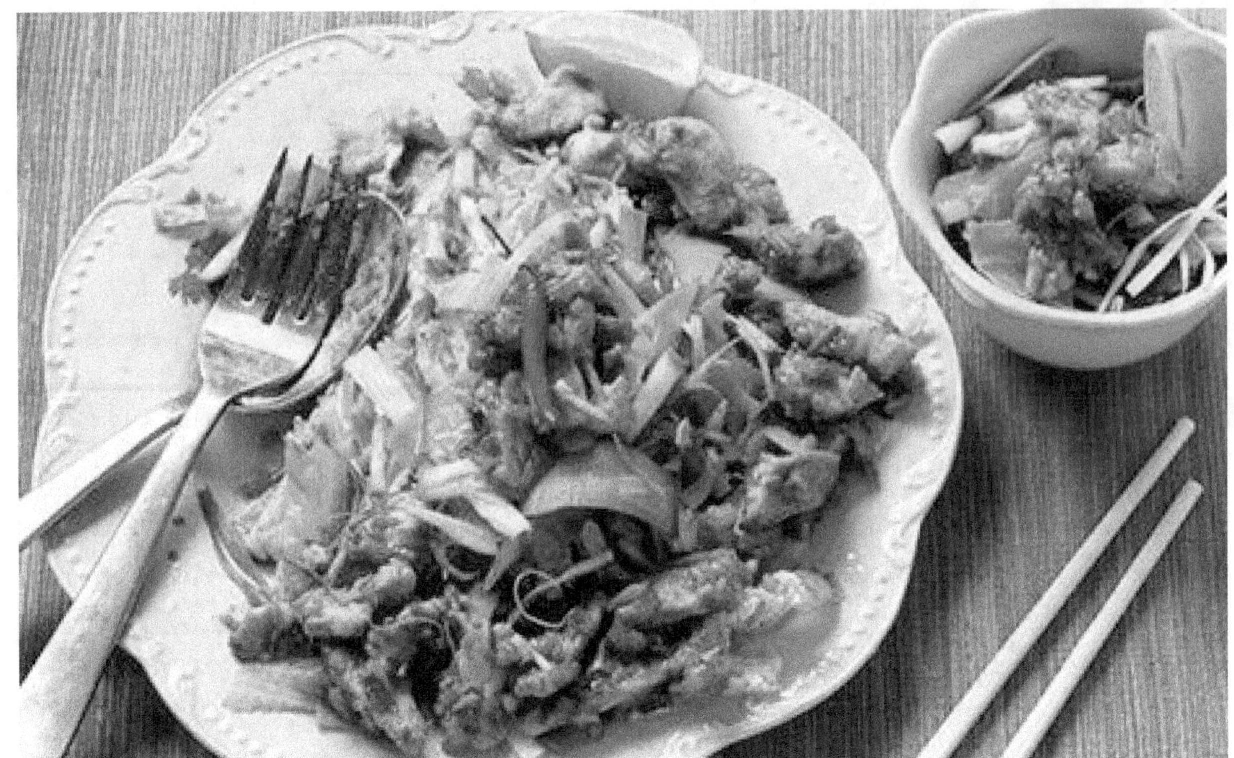

Breakfast: Wholemeal toast with grilled bacon and mushrooms

Lunch: Bang bang chicken salad

Dinner: Coq au vin with Broccoli

Pudding: Hot chocolate

Choose from snacks, including raspberry smoothie and nuts.

Sunday's low-carb meal plan

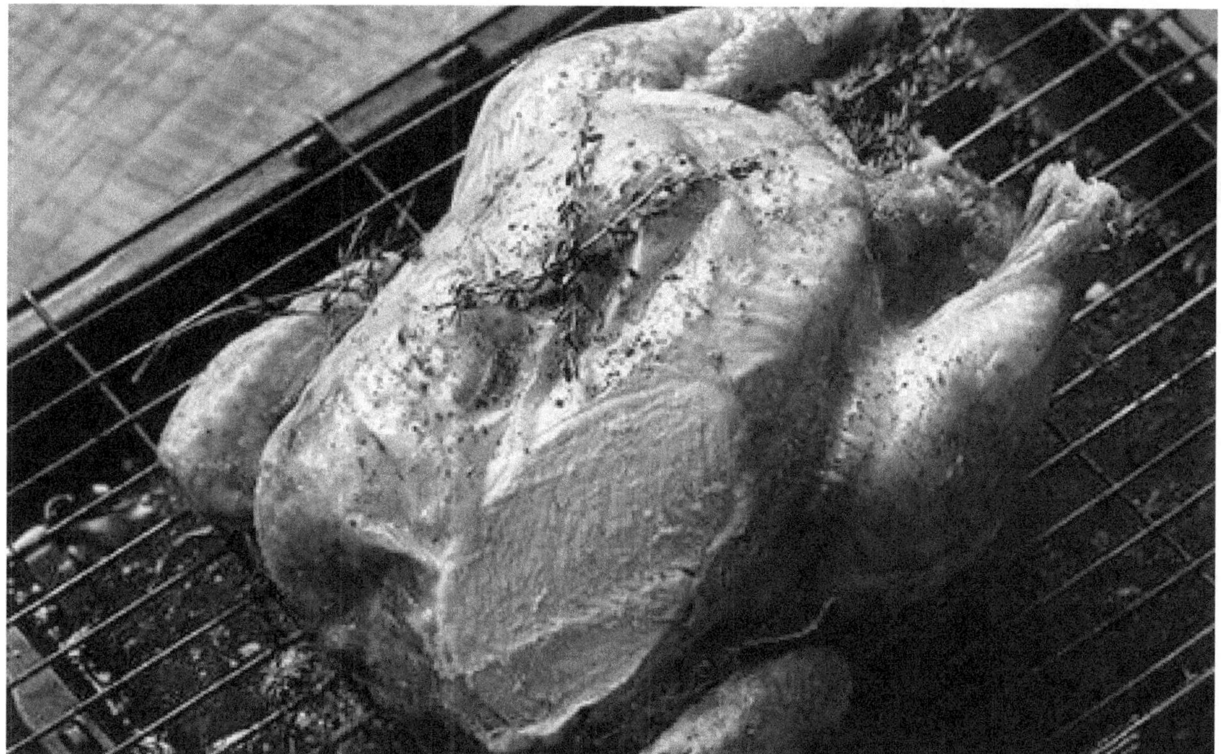

Breakfast: Scrambled egg with smoked salmon on granary toast

Lunch: Ham, leek, and Parmesan frittata with avocado, celery, cucumber, and lettuce

Dinner: Roast chicken, roast potatoes, green beans, and gravy

Pudding: Greek Yogurt with raspberries

Choose from snacks, including olives, nuts, dried fruit, and oatcakes with light cream cheese.

BENEFITS OF FOLLOWING A LOW-CARB DIET

One of the main benefits of following a low-carb diet is weight loss. For people with type 2 diabetes, this helps to reduce HbA1c and blood fats such as cholesterol. For people who don't have diabetes, losing weight can reduce your risk of developing type 2 diabetes, and a low-carb diet is one option to lose weight.

For people with type 1 diabetes

If you have type 1, it's essential to know that the best way to keep your blood sugar levels steady is to carb count rather than following a particular diet. And there is no substantial evidence that following a low-carb diet is safe or beneficial, which is why we don't recommend this diet for people with type 1 diabetes. But some people with type 1 have reported needing less insulin and losing weight from following a low-carb diet.

You must speak to your healthcare team for support to manage your insulin if you're considering a low-carb diet.

For people with type 2 diabetes

If you have type 2 diabetes, our research has shown that losing around 15kg within three to five months significantly improves your chances of putting your type 2 diabetes into remission.

Research funded by an American company also found that some people with type 2 diabetes who followed a program that included a low-carb eating plan were in remission after two years. Participants in the study were supported to restrict their intake of carbs, initially to less than 30g per day and then gradually increasing the amount, based on personal tolerance and health goals.

If you have obesity, finding a way to lose weight can also reduce your risk of complications. There are different ways of doing this, and a low-carb diet is one option.

However, there's no evidence that following a low-carb diet is more beneficial in managing diabetes than other approaches in the long term, including a healthy, balanced diet. Research suggests that the best type of diet is one that you can maintain in the long term, so it's important to talk to your healthcare professional about what you think will work for you. Another option is the Mediterranean diet, which is also linked to reducing the risk of heart diseases and stroke.

WHAT TO CONSIDER BEFORE FOLLOWING A LOW-CARB DIET

If you treat your diabetes with insulin or any other medication that puts you at risk of hypos (low blood sugar levels), following a low-carb diet may increase this risk. Speak to your healthcare team about this so they can help you adjust your medications to reduce your risk of hypos. Your team may also support you to check your blood sugar levels more often.

Depending on the approach, following a low-carb diet may also lead to other side effects, such as constipation or bad breath. Although these can be unpleasant, they are usually temporary and shouldn't be harmful in the long term. Speak to your healthcare professional if you're concerned about any of these.

It's essential to first reduce your carb intake from unhealthy sources such as sugary drinks, pizzas, cakes, biscuits, chips, white bread, fruit juices, and smoothies. And it is a good idea to get your limited carbs from healthy high-fiber carb foods, such as pulses, nuts, vegetables, whole fruits, and whole grains, as well as unsweetened milk and Yogurt.

DIABETES: BEST DIETS FOR WEIGHT LOSS

For people with diabetes, reaching and maintaining a healthy weight is essential. A healthy weight helps manage blood sugar levels and reduce the chances of additional complications, such as a stroke or heart attack.

People with diabetes who want to lose weight must do so safely. Trying to lose weight too fast or being too restrictive can also lead to blood sugar levels. Obesity is a risk factor for type 2 diabetes. It is also becoming more common in people with type 1 diabetes.

A person with diabetes must consider several factors when deciding on the best way to lose weight. Factors to consider include their age, general health, and how much weight they have to lose. It is best to talk to a healthcare professional before starting any new weight-loss plan.

The best weight-loss diet for someone with diabetes is one they will stick to long-term. The following diets involve making beneficial long-term changes to help a person lose weight safely:

Mediterranean Diet

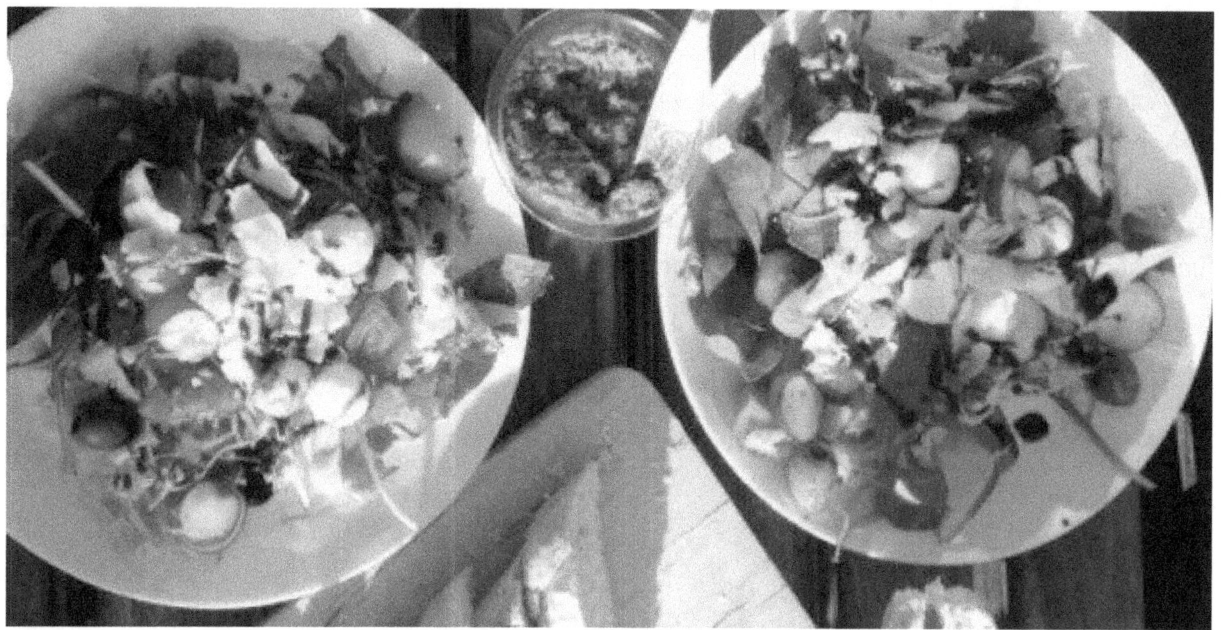

The Mediterranean diet involves food choices and cooking styles typical of some places in the Mediterranean region.

The diet includes:

- Plenty Of Vegetables
- Whole Grains
- Fruits In Moderation
- Nuts And Seeds
- Herbs And Spices
- Olive Oil
- Fish
- Eggs

The authors of a 2017 review noted that the Mediterranean diet might be a useful approach to weight loss for people with diabetes.

They highlighted a 2-year study that involved 36 adults with obesity and types 2 diabetes. The participants ate either a low-carbohydrate diet, a Mediterranean diet, or a low-fat diet for two years.

The Mediterranean diet was the most favorable for changes in insulin and fasting glucose levels. Those following the Mediterranean diet also lost an average of 1.5 kilograms (kg), or 3.3 pounds more than those on a low-fat diet.

Low-Carb Diet

Low-carb diets are a popular weight loss plan. Typically, low-carb diets limit a person's carbohydrate intake and include higher amounts of protein and healthful fats.

Examples of foods that to avoid on a low-carb diet include:

- Potatoes
- Rice
- White Bread
- Cakes
- Sweets
- Bagels
- Pasta

People on a low-carb diet should eat plenty of vegetables and get lots of protein from fish, lean meats, and eggs. To learn more about what to eat on a low-carb diet.Some studies show that low-carb diets may be effective and safe for people who have diabetes.

One study involved adults who had prediabetes or type 2 diabetes and had a body mass index (BMI) over 25.

The study participants ate either a very low-carb, high-fat, non-calorie restriction diet, a medium-carb, low-fat, calorie-restricted diet.

After three months, the group on the low-carb, high-fat diet lost 5.5 kg (about 12 pounds), compared to a 2.6 kg (5.7 pounds) weight loss for those following the medium-carb low-fat diet.

Additionally, 44% of those on the low-carb diet discontinued at least one diabetes medication.

It is vital to realize that there are different versions of low-carb diets. Some diets restrict carbohydrates to as low as 20 grams (g) or less per day, which may not be suitable for everyone.

Paleolithic Diet

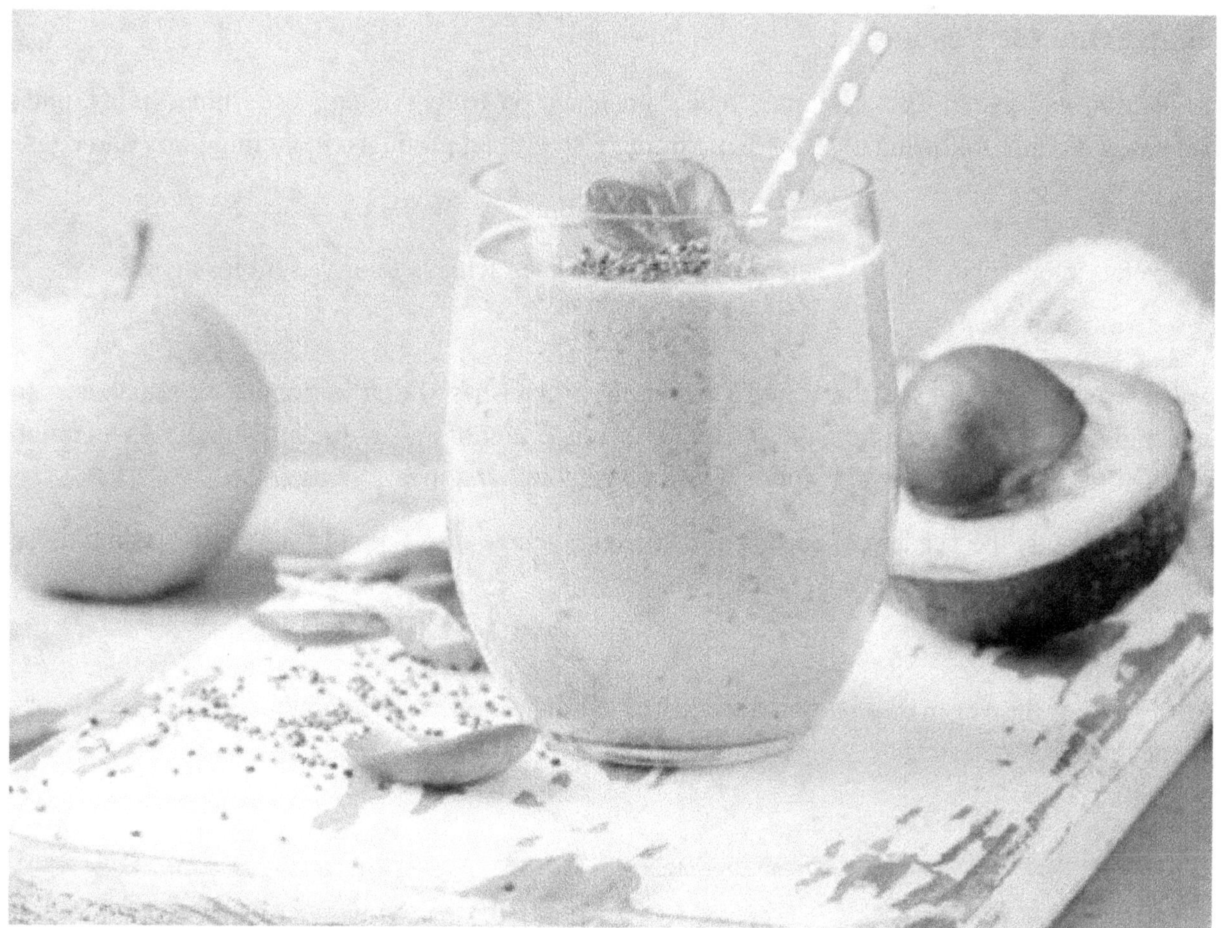

Fruits and vegetables are an everyday staple of weight-loss diets.

The Paleolithic or "paleo" diet attempts to replicate the diet that people ate thousands of years ago when hunting for food. Staples of a paleolithic diet include fruits, vegetables, lean meat, and fish.

Many of the foods included in the paleo diet are similar to those in a low-carb diet, as a paleo diet prohibits most grains' consumption.

In a small 2013 study, 13 people with type 2 diabetes followed the paleo diet for three months, then switched to a diabetic diet for three months.

The diabetic diet included evenly distributed meals that contained dietary FiberFiber, whole grain bread, cereals, and vegetables. The researchers found that the paleo diet was more filling per calorie than the diabetic diet. Participants noticed greater weight loss with the paleo diet but found it more challenging to sustain.

Vegetarian Or Vegan

Vegetarian and vegan diets eliminate meat and focus on fruits, vegetables, whole grains, nuts, and seeds. People following a vegan diet eliminate all animal products, including dairy and eggs.

A vegetarian or vegan diet may help people with diabetes achieve their weight loss goals.

A 2017 review highlighted the benefits of eating a plant-based diet in people with diabetes. In one study, 99 people of varying ages ate either a vegan diet or an American Diabetic Association (ADA) diet that included whole grains, fruits, vegetables, and meat.

After 22 weeks, the vegan diet participants lost an average of 6.5 kg (14.3 pounds), while those on the ADA diet lost 3.1 kg (6.8 pounds).

Also, 43% of the vegan diet participants decreased their diabetic medications, compared to 26% on the ADA diet.

5-DAY DIABETES MEAL PLAN FOR WEIGHT LOSS

Lose weight and keep your blood sugar steady with this healthy 5-day diabetes diet meal plan. Each of the five days offers healthy meals and snacks balanced for carbohydrates, protein, and FiberFiber to help keep your blood sugar steady as you cut calories to lose weight. Each meal contains 2-3 carb servings (30-45 grams of carbohydrates), and each snack is around 1 carb serving (15 grams of carbohydrates). Aim to keep your daily calorie total at 1,500 calories, which will put you on track to lose a healthy 1 to 2 pounds per week. We kept the days in this plan slightly under 1,500 calories so you'd have the freedom to add in a beverage of your choice or a diabetes-friendly dessert. And don't forget to stay hydrated! Aim for 64 oz. of water every day. With the healthy meals and snacks in this plan, losing weight with diabetes is a delicious and straightforward endeavor.

DAY 1

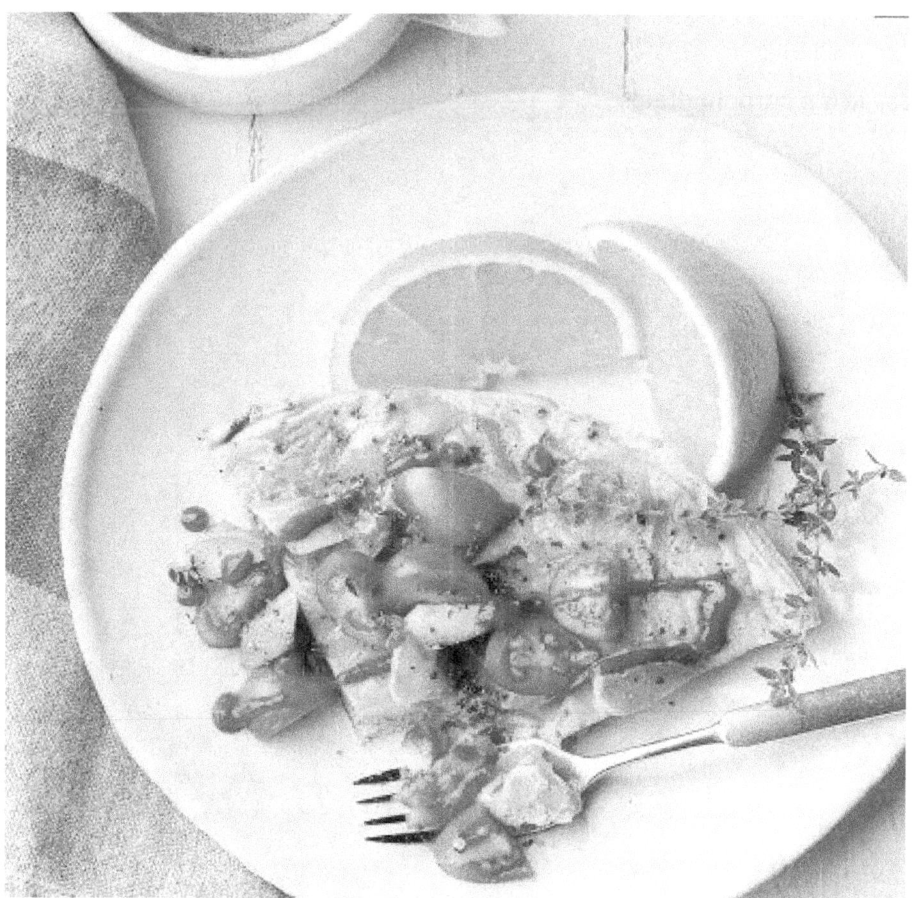

Breakfast

- 1 serving rainbow Frittata
- 1 slice whole-wheat toast

- 1 Tbsp. reduced-sugar jelly

Snack

- 1 medium banana
- 1 Tbsp. peanut butter

Lunch

- 1 serving Spicy Thai Noodles

Snack

- 1 low-fat cheese stick
- 1 cup raspberries

Dinner

- 1 serving Greek Chicken with Roasted Spring Vegetables

Daily Total: 1,359 calories, 136 g carbohydrates

DAY 2

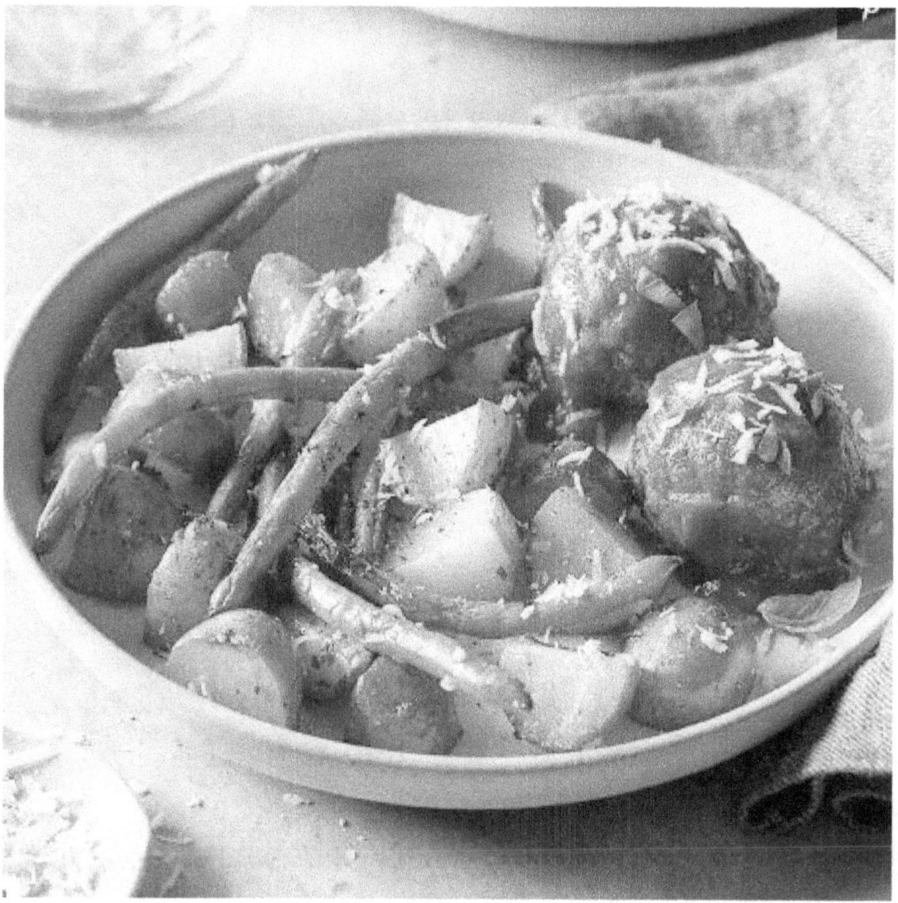

Breakfast

- 1 whole-wheat English muffin half
- 1/4 avocado, mashed
- 1 over-easy egg
- 1/2 cup grapes

Snack

- 2 Tbsp. raisins
- 2 Tbsp. unsalted peanuts

Lunch

- 1 serving Strawberry Arugula Salad
- 6 oz. light vanilla Greek Yogurt

Snack

- 1/4 cup hummus
- 1 cup carrot sticks

Dinner

- 1 serving Meatballs with Roasted Green Beans and Potatoes
- 1 cup raspberries

Daily Total: 1,244 calories, 146 g carbohydrates

DAY 3

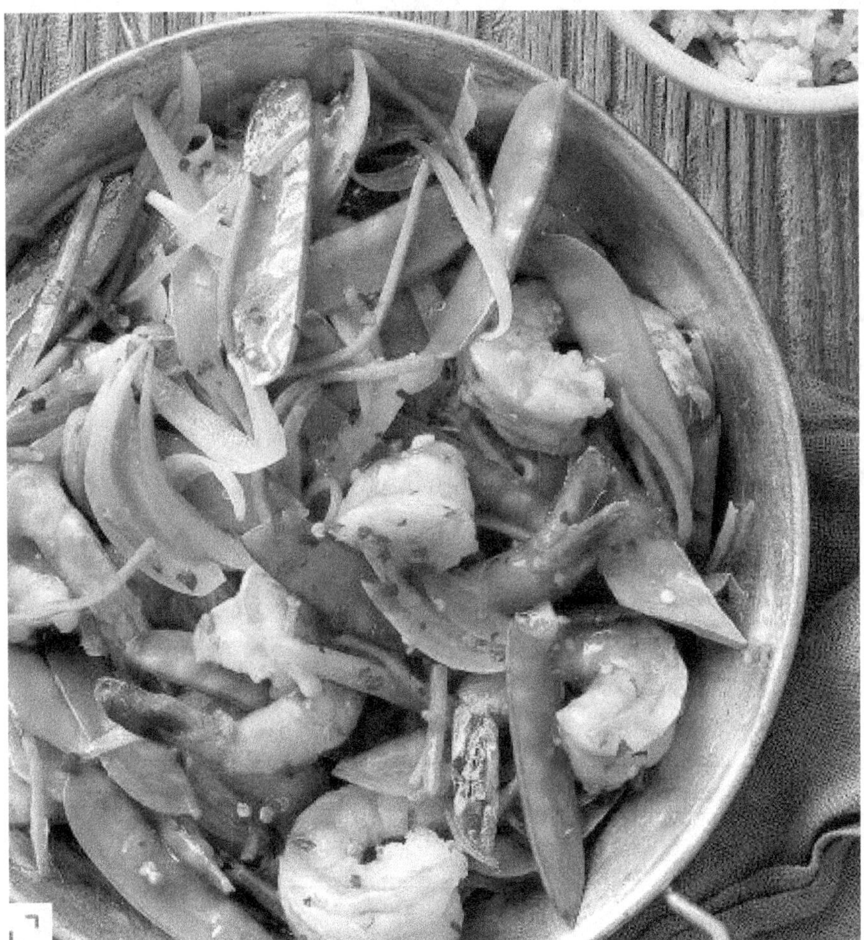

Breakfast

- 1 hard-cooked egg
- 1 serving Cherry-Mocha Smoothie

Snack

- 1 wedge light Swiss spreadable cheese
- 7 reduced-fat wheat crackers

- 1/2 cup grapes

Lunch

- 1 servingSpringtime Cacio e Pepe
- 1 cup carrot sticks
- 1 Tbsp. light ranch dressing

Snack

- 2 Tbsp. raisins
- 2 Tbsp. unsalted peanuts

Dinner

- 1 serving Shrimp and Pea Pod Stir-Fry
- 1 cup whole strawberries

Daily Total: 1,336 calories, 160 g carbohydrates

DAY 4

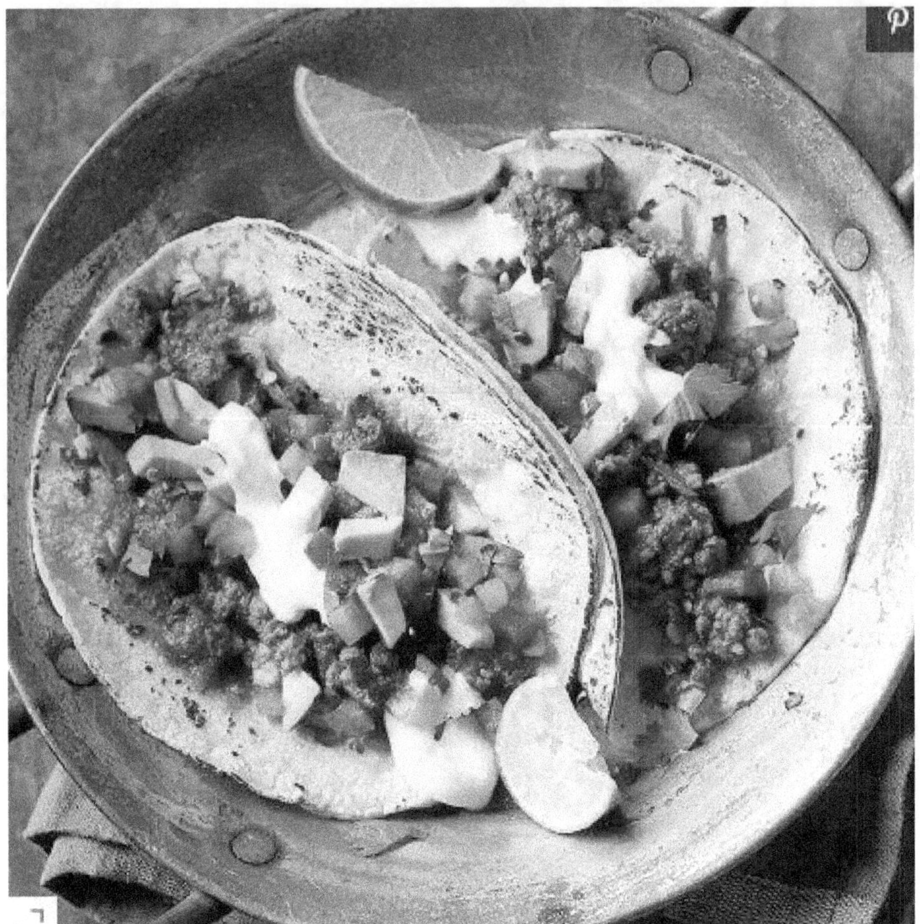

Breakfast

- 1 whole-wheat English muffin half
- 1/4 avocado, mashed
- 1 over-easy egg
- 1/2 cup grapes

Snack

- 1 cup carrot sticks
- 1 Tbsp. light ranch dressing

Lunch

- 1 serving Thai-Style Salad
- 1 medium banana

Snack

- 1/4 cup hummus
- 1 cup green bell pepper strips

Dinner

- 1 serving Chipotle Beef Tacos
- 1 serving Mexican Street Corn
- 1 serving Tangy Pepper Salad

Daily Total: 1,389 calories, 162 g carbohydrates

DAY 5

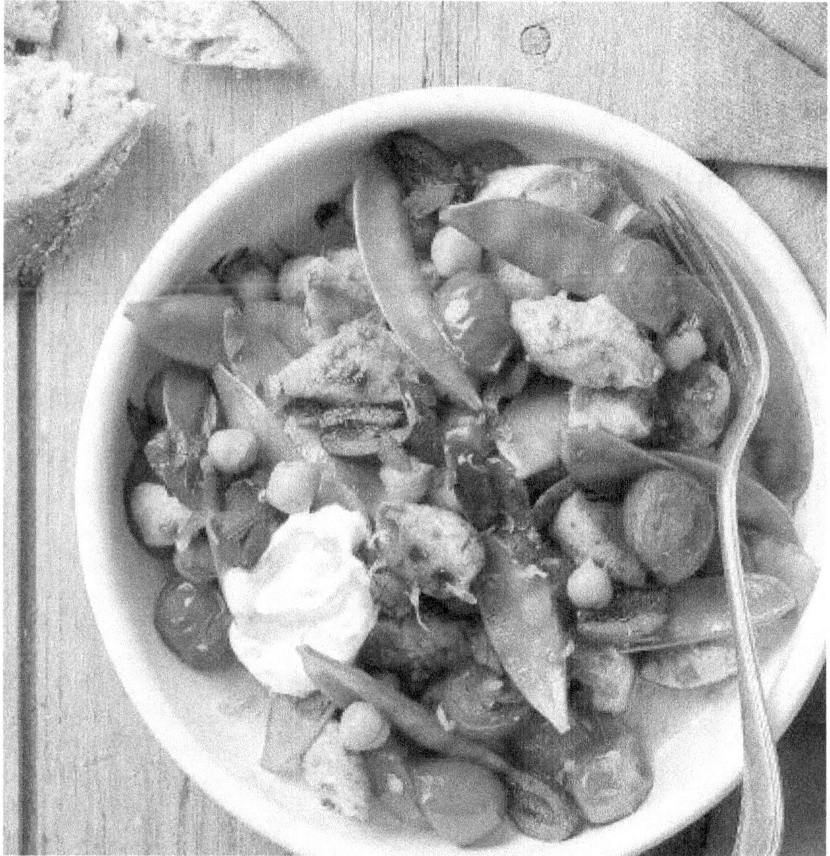

Breakfast

- 1 cup oatmeal (prepared with water)
- 1 Tbsp. peanut butter
- 1/2 cup blueberries

Snack

- 1 cup grapes

- 1 low-fat mozzarella cheese stick

Lunch

- 1 serving Bacon Ranch Salad
- 1 cup whole strawberries

Snack

- 2 Tbsp. raisins
- 2 Tbsp. unsalted peanuts

Dinner

- 1 serving Spicy Chicken and Snow Pea Skillet
- 1 cup raspberries

Daily Total: 1,288 calories, 142 g carbohydrates

DIABETIC COOKING COOKBOOK

Finding tasty diabetes recipes can be challenging. This Diabetes Cookbook provides delicious recipes for cooking .

CONDIMENTS

Basil Pesto

- ❖ 1 cup basil
- ❖ 1/3 cup cashews
- ❖ 2 garlic cloves, chopped
- ❖ 1/2 cup olive oil or avocado oil Process basil, cashews, and garlic until smooth.

- ● Add oil in a slow stream. The process to combine.
- ● Transfer to a bowl.
- ● Season with salt and pepper.
- ● Stir to combine.

Allergies: SF, GF, DF, EF, V

Cilantro Pesto

- ❖ 1 cup cilantro
- ❖ 1/3 cup cashews
- ❖ 2 garlic cloves, chopped
- ❖ 1/2 cup olive oil or avocado oil Process cilantro, cashews, and garlic.

- ● Add oil in a slow stream. The process to combine.
- ● Transfer to a bowl.

- Season with salt and pepper.
- Stir to combine.

Allergies: SF, GF, DF, EF, V

Sundried Tomato Pesto

- ❖ 3/4 cup sundried tomatoes
- ❖ 1/3 cup cashews
- ❖ 2 garlic cloves, chopped
- ❖ 1/2 cup olive oil or cumin oil Process tomato, cashews, and garlic.

- Add oil in a slow stream. The process to combine.
- Transfer to a bowl.
- Season with salt and pepper.
- Stir to combine.

Allergies: SF, GF, DF, EF, V

BROTHS

Some recipes require a cup or more of various broths, vegetables, Beef, or chicken broth. I usually cook the whole pot and freeze it.

Vegetable broth

Servings: 6 cups Ingredients

- ❖ 1 tbsp. coconut oil
- ❖ 1 large onion
- ❖ 2 stalks celery, including some leaves
- ❖ 2 large carrots
- ❖ 1 bunch green onions, chopped
- ❖ 8 cloves garlic, minced
- ❖ 8 sprigs fresh parsley
- ❖ 6 sprigs fresh thyme
- ❖ 2 bay leaves
- ❖ 1 tsp. salt
- ❖ 2 quarts of water

Allergies: SF, GF, DF, EF, V, NF

Instructions

- Chop veggies into small chunks.
- Heat oil in a soup pot and add onion, scallions, celery, carrots, garlic, parsley, thyme, and bay leaves.
- Cook over high heat for 5 to 7 minutes, stirring occasionally.
- Bring to a boil and add salt.
- Lower heat and simmer, uncovered, for 30 minutes. Strain.
- Other ingredients to consider: broccoli stalk, celery root

Chicken Broth

Ingredients

- ❖ 4 lbs. fresh ChickenChicken (wings, necks, backs, legs, bones)
- ❖ 2 peeled onions or 1 cup chopped leeks
- ❖ 2 celery stalks
- ❖ 1 carrot
- ❖ 8 black peppercorns
- ❖ 2 sprigs fresh thyme
- ❖ 2 sprigs fresh parsley
- ❖ 1 tsp. salt Instructions –

Allergies: SF, GF, DF, EF, NF

- Put cold water in a stockpot and add ChickenChicken.
- Bring just to a boil.
- Skim any foam from the surface.
- Add other ingredients, return just to a boil, and reduce heat to a slow simmer.
- Simmer for 2 hours.
- Let cool to warm room temperature and strain.
- Keep chilled and use or freeze broth within a few days.
- Before using, defrost, and boil.

Beef Broth

Ingredients

- ❖ 4-5 pounds beef bones and few veal bones
- ❖ 1 pound of stew meat (chuck or flank steak) cut into 2-inch chunks
- ❖ Olive oil
- ❖ 1-2 medium onions, peeled and quartered
- ❖ 1-2 large carrots, cut into 1-2 inch segments   1 celery rib, cut into 1-inch segments

- ❖ 2-3 cloves of garlic, unpeeled
- ❖ Handful of parsley stems and leaves
- ❖ 1-2 bay leaves
- ❖ 10 peppercorns

Allergies: SF, GF, DF, EF, NF

Instructions -

- Heat oven to 375°F. Rub olive oil over the stew meat pieces, carrots, and onions.
- Place stew meat or beef scraps, stock bones, carrots, and onions in a large roasting pan.
- Roast in the oven for about 45 minutes, turning everything halfway through the cooking.
- Place everything from the oven in a large stockpot.
- Pour some boiling water in the oven pan and scrape up all of the browned bits, and pour all in the stockpot.
- Add parsley, celery, garlic, bay leaves, and peppercorns to the pot.
- Fill the pot with cold water to 1 inch over the top of the bones.
- Bring the stockpot to a steady simmer and then reduce the heat to low, so it just barely simmers.
- Cover the pot loosely and let simmer low and slow for 3-4 hours.
- Scoop away the fat and any scum that rises to the surface once in a while.
- After cooking, remove the bones and vegetables from the pot. Strain the broth.
- Let cool to room temperature and then put in the refrigerator.
- The fat will solidify once the broth has chilled. Discard the fat (or reuse it) and pour the broth into a jar and freeze it.

PASTES

Curry Paste

This should not be prepared in advance, but several curry recipes are using curry paste, and I decided to make the curry paste recipe out and have it separately.

When you see that the recipe uses curry paste, please go to this part of the book and prepare it from scratch.

Don't use processed curry pastes or curry powder; make it every time from scratch. Keep the original form(seeds, pods), ground them just before making the curry paste. You can dry heat in the skillet cloves, cardamom, cumin, and coriander and then crush them coarsely with mortar and pestle.

Ingredients

- 2 onions, minced
- 2 cloves garlic, minced
- 2 teaspoons fresh ginger root, finely chopped
- 6 whole cloves
- 2 cardamom pods
- 2 (2 inch) pieces cinnamon sticks, crushed
- 1 tsp. ground cumin
- 1 tsp. ground coriander
- 1 tsp. salt
- 1 tsp. ground cayenne pepper
- 1 tsp. ground turmeric

Allergies: SF, GF, DF, EF, V, NF

Instructions -

- Heat oil in a frying pan over medium heat and fry onions until transparent.
- Stir in garlic, cumin, ginger, cloves, cinnamon, coriander, salt, cayenne, and turmeric.
- Cook for 1 minute over medium heat, stirring constantly.
- At this point, other curry ingredients should be added.

Tomato paste

Some recipes (chili) require tomato paste. I usually prepare 20 or so liters at once (when the tomato is in season, which is usually September) and freeze it.

Ingredients

- 5 lbs. chopped plump tomatoes
- 1/4 cup extra-virgin olive oil or avocado oil plus 2 tbsp.
- salt, to taste

Allergies: SF, GF, DF, EF, V, NF

Instructions –

- Heat 1/4 cup of the oil in a skillet over medium heat.
- Add tomatoes.
- Season with salt. Bring to a boil.
- Cook, stirring, until very soft, about 8 minutes.
- Pass the tomatoes through the most pleasing plate of a food mill.
- Push as much of the pulp through the sieve as possible and leave the seeds behind.
- Bring it to boil, lower it and then boil uncovered so that the liquid will thicken (approx. 30-40 minutes). That will give you homemade tomato juice.
- You get tomato paste if you boil for 60 minutes; it gets thick like store-bought ketchup.
- Store sealed in an airtight container in the refrigerator for up to one month, or freeze for up to 6 months.

Precooked beans

Some recipes also require that you cook some beans (butter beans, red kidney, garbanzo) in advance. Cooking beans takes around 3 hours, and it can be done in advance or every few weeks, and the rest gets frozen. Soak beans for 24 hours before cooking them. After the first boil, throw the water, add new water, and continue cooking. Some beans or lentils can be sprouted a few days before cooking, helping people with stomach problems.

BREAKFAST - OATMEAL

Oatmeal Breakfast

Allergies: SF, GF, DF, EF, V, NF

- ❖ 1/2 cup dry oatmeal
- ❖ 2 tsp. Of ground flax seeds
- ❖ 2 tsp. of sunflower seeds
- ❖ A dash of cinnamon
- ❖ 1 tsp. of cocoa

- ● Cook oatmeal with hot water, and after that, mix all ingredients.
- ● Sweeten if you have to with few drops of lucuma powder.
- ● **Optional:** You can replace sunflower seeds with pumpkin seeds or chia seeds.
- ● You can add a handful of blueberries or any berries instead of cocoa.

Oatmeal Yogurt Breakfast

Allergies: SF, GF, EF, NF

- ❖ 1/2 cup dry oatmeal
- ❖ Handful of blueberries (optional)
- ❖ 1 cups of low-fat Yogurt

Mix all ingredients and wait 20 minutes or leave overnight in the fridge if using steel cut oats

Cocoa Oatmeal

Allergies: SF, GF, DF, NF

Ingredients

- ❖ 1/2 cup dry oats
- ❖ 1 cup of water
- ❖ A pinch tsp. salt
- ❖ 1/2 tsp. ground vanilla bean
- ❖ 1 tbsp. cocoa powder
- ❖ 1 tbsp. lucuma powder
- ❖ 3 tbsp. ground flax seeds meal
- ❖ a dash of cinnamon
- ❖ 2 egg whites

Instructions

- In a saucepan over high heat, place the oats and salt.
- Cover with water.
- Bring to a boil and cook for 3-5 minutes, stirring occasionally.
- Keep adding 1/2 cup water if necessary as the mixture thickens.
- In a separate bowl, whisk 4 tbsp. Water into the 1 tbsp. Cocoa powder to form a smooth sauce.
- Add the vanilla to the pan and stir.
- Turn the heat down to Low.
- Add the egg whites and whisk immediately.
- Add the flax meal and cinnamon.
- Stir to combine.
- Remove from heat, add lucuma powder, and serve immediately.
- Topping suggestions: sliced strawberries, blueberries, or a few almonds.

Flax and Blueberry Vanilla Overnight Oats

Allergies: SF, GF, EF, V, NF

Ingredients –

- ❖ 1/2 cup dry oats
- ❖ 1/3 cup water
- ❖ 1/2 cup low-fat Yogurt
- ❖ 1/2 tsp. Ground vanilla bean
- ❖ 2 tbsp. flax seeds meal

- ❖ A pinch of salt
- ❖ Blueberries, almonds, blackberries, lucuma powder for topping

Instructions

- Add the ingredients (except for toppings) to the bowl in the evening.
- Refrigerate overnight.
- In the morning, stir up the mixture.
- It should be thick.
- Add the toppings of your choice.

Apple Oatmeal

Allergies: SF, GF, DF, EF, V, NF

Ingredients -

- ❖ 1/2 grated apple
- ❖ 1/2 cup dry oats
- ❖ 1 cups water
- ❖ Dash of cinnamon
- ❖ 1 tsp. lucuma powder Instructions

- Cook the oats with the water for 3-5 minutes.
- Add grated apple and cinnamon.
- Stir in the lucuma powder.

Coconut Pomegranate Oatmeal

Allergies: SF, GF, DF, EF, V, NF

Ingredients -

- 1/2 cup dry oats
- 1/3 cup coconut milk
- 1 cups water
- 2 tbs. shredded unsweetened coconut
- 1 tbs. flax seeds meal
- 1 tbs. lucuma powder
- 4 tbs. pomegranate seeds

Instructions

- Cook oats with coconut milk, water, and salt.
- Stir in the coconut, lucuma powder, and flaxseed meal.
- Sprinkle with extra coconut and pomegranate seeds.

<h1 align="center">SAVORY BREAKFASTS</h1>

Omelet with Leeks

Allergies: SF, GF, DF, NF

Cook 1 cup chopped leeks in little coconut oil until they get soft, and then mix the 2 beaten eggs.

Egg pizza crust

Allergies: SF, GF, DF, NF

Ingredients -

- ❖ 2 eggs
- ❖ 1/4 cup of coconut flour
- ❖ 1/2 cup of coconut milk
- ❖ 1 small crushed garlic clove

- ● Mix and make an omelet.

Omelet with veggies

Allergies: SF, GF, DF, NF

Ingredients -

- ❖ 2 large eggs
- ❖ Salt
- ❖ Ground black pepper
- ❖ 1 tsp. olive oil or cumin oil
- ❖ 1cups spinach, cherry tomatoes, and 1 spoon of yogurt cheese

* ❖ Crushed red
* ❖ pepper flakes and a pinch of dill (optional)

Instructions

* Whisk 2 large eggs in a bowl.
* Season with salt and ground black pepper and set aside.
* Heat 1 tsp. Olive oil in a medium skillet over medium heat.
* Add baby spinach, tomatoes, cheese, and cook, tossing, until wilted (approx. 1 minute).
* Add eggs; cook, occasionally stirring, until just set, about 1 minute.
* Stir in cheese.
* Sprinkle with crushed red pepper flakes and dill.

Egg Muffins

Allergies: SF, GF, DF, NF

Serving: 4 muffins

Ingredients -

* ❖ 4 eggs
* ❖ 1/2 cup diced green bell pepper
* ❖ 1/2 cup diced onion
* ❖ 1/2 cup Spinach
* ❖ 1/4 tsp. salt
* ❖ 1/8 tsp. ground black pepper
* ❖ 2 tbsp. water

Instructions

* Heat the oven to 350 degrees F. Oil 4 muffin cups.
* Beat eggs together.

- Mix in bell pepper, Spinach, onion, salt, black pepper, and water.
- Pour the mixture into muffin cups.
- Bake in the oven until muffins are done in the middle.

Smoked Salmon Scrambled Eggs

Allergies: SF, GF, DF, NF

Ingredients -

- 1 tsp coconut oil
- 2 eggs
- 1 Tbs water
- 2 oz smoked salmon, sliced
- 1/4 avocado
- ground black pepper, to taste
- 2 chives, minced (or use 1 green onion, thinly sliced)

Instructions

- Heat a skillet over medium heat.
- Add coconut oil to the pan when hot.
- Meanwhile, scramble eggs.
- Add eggs to the hot skillet, along with smoked salmon.
- Stirring continuously, cook eggs until soft and fluffy.
- Remove from heat.
- Top with avocado, black pepper, and chives to serve.

Steak and Eggs

Allergies: SF, GF, DF, NF

Ingredients -

- ❖ 1/4 lb boneless beef steak or pork tenderloin • 1/4 tsp ground black pepper
- ❖ 1/4 tsp sea salt (optional)
- ❖ 1 tsp coconut oil
- ❖ 1/4 onion, diced
- ❖ 1/2 red bell pepper, diced
- ❖ 1 handful spinach or arugula
- ❖ 1 egg Instructions

- Season sliced steak or pork tenderloin with sea salt and black pepper.
- Heat a sauté pan over high heat.
- Add 1 tsp coconut oil, onions, and meat when the pan is hot, and sauté until the steak is slightly cooked.
- Add spinach and red bell pepper, and cook until steak is done to your liking.
- Meanwhile, heat a small frypan over medium heat.
- Add remaining coconut oil, and fry two eggs.
- Top steak with a fried egg to serve.

Egg Bake

Allergies: SF, GF, DF, NF

Ingredients -

- ❖ 1/2 cup chopped red peppers or Spinach
- ❖ 1/4 cup zucchini
- ❖ 1/2 tbsp. coconut oil

❖ 1/4 cup sliced green onions

❖ 2 eggs

❖ 1/4 cup coconut milk

❖ 1/8 cup almond flour

❖ 1 tbsp. Minced fresh parsley

❖ 1/4 tsp. dried basil

❖ 1/8 tsp. salt

❖ 1/8 tsp. ground black pepper

Instructions

● Preheat oven to 350 degrees F.

● Put coconut oil in a skillet.

● Heat it to medium heat.

● Add mushrooms, onions, zucchini, and red pepper (or Spinach) until vegetables are tender, about 5 minutes.

● Drain veggies and spread them over the baking dish.

● Beat eggs in a bowl with milk, flour, parsley, basil, salt, and pepper.

● Pour egg mixture into baking dish.

● Bake in the preheated oven until the center is set (approx. 35 to 40 minutes).

Frittata

Allergies: SF, GF, DF, NF

Ingredients -

❖ 1 tbsp. olive oil or avocado oil

❖ 1/2 Zucchini, sliced

❖ 1/4 cup torn fresh Spinach

❖ 1 tbsp. sliced green onions

❖ 1/4 tsp. crushed garlic, salt, and pepper to taste

❖ 1/8 cup coconut milk

❖ 2 eggs Instructions

- Heat olive oil in a skillet over medium heat.
- Add zucchini and cook until tender.
- Mix in Spinach, green onions, and Garlic.
- Season with salt and pepper. Continue cooking until Spinach is wilted.
- In a separate bowl, beat together eggs and coconut milk.
- Pour into the skillet over the vegetables.
- Reduce heat to low, cover, and cook until eggs are firm (5 to 7 minutes).

Naan Pancakes Crepes

Allergies: SF, GF, DF, EF, V

Ingredients -

❖ 1/2 cup almond flour

❖ 1/2 cup Tapioca Flour

❖ 1 cup Coconut Milk

❖ Salt

❖ coconut oil

❖ Instructions

- Mix all the ingredients.
- Heat a pan over medium heat and pour batter to desired thickness.
- Once the batter looks firm, flip it over to cook the other side.
- If you want this to be a dessert crepe or pancake, then omit the salt.
- You can add minced garlic or ginger in the batter if you want, or some spices.

Zucchini Pancakes

Allergies: SF, GF, DF

Ingredients -

- ❖ 1 small zucchini
- ❖ 1 tbsp. Chopped onion
- ❖ 2 beaten eggs
- ❖ 3 tbsp. Almond flour
- ❖ 1/2 tsp. salt
- ❖ 1/2 tsp. ground black pepper
- ❖ coconut oil

Instructions

- ● Heat the oven to 300 degrees F.
- ● Grate the zucchini into a bowl and stir in the onion and eggs.
- ● Stir in 6 tbsp. of the flour, salt, and pepper.
- ● Heat a large sauté pan over medium heat and add coconut oil to the pan.
- ● When the oil is hot, lower the heat to medium-low and add batter into the pan.
- ● Cook the pancakes for about 2 minutes on each side, until browned.
- ● Place the pancakes in the oven.

Smoothies

Put the liquid in first. Surrounded by tea or Yogurt, the blender blades can move freely. Next, add chunks of fruits or vegetables. Leafy greens are going into the pitcher last. The preferred liquid is green tea, but you can use almond or coconut milk or herbal tea.

Start slow. If your blender has sped, start it on Low to break up big pieces of fruit. Continue blending until you get a puree. If your blender can pulse, pulse a few times before switching to a puree mode. Once you have your liquid and fruit pureed, start adding greens, very slowly. Wait until the previous batch of greens has been thoroughly blended.

Thicken? Added too much tea or coconut milk? Thicken your smoothie by adding ice cubes, flax meal, chia seeds, or oatmeal. Once you get used to smoothies' various tastes, add any seaweed, spirulina, chlorella powder, or ginger for an additional kick. Think of adding any nut butter or sesame paste too or some oils.

Rotate! Rotate your greens; don't always drink the same smoothie! In the beginning, try 2 different greens every week and later introduce the third and fourth one weekly. And keep rotating them. Don't use Spinach and Kale all the time.

Try beets greens; they have a pinch of pink in them, which adds great color to your smoothie. Here is the list of leafy green for you to try: Spinach, Kale, dandelion, chards, beet leaves, arugula, lettuce, collard greens, bok choy, cabbage, cilantro, parsley.

Flavor! Flavor smoothies with ground vanilla bean, cinnamon, lucuma powder, nutmeg, cloves, almond butter, cayenne pepper, ginger, or just about any seeds or chopped nuts combination.

Not only are green smoothies high in nutrients, vitamins, and fiber, they can also make any vegetable you probably don't like (be it kale, spinach, or broccoli) taste great.

 The secret behind blending the perfect smoothie is using sweet fruits or nuts, or seeds to give your drink a unique taste. There's a reason kale and spinach seem to be the main ingredients in almost every green smoothie.

Not only do they give smoothies their green color, but they are also packed with calcium, protein, and iron. Although blending alone increases the accessibility of carotenoids, since fats are known to increase carotenoid absorption from leafy greens, it is possible that coconut oil, nuts, and seeds in a smoothie could increase absorption further. If you can't find some ingredient, replace it with the closest one.

GREEN SMOOTHIES

Kale Kiwi Smoothie

- ❖ 1 cup Kale, chopped
- ❖ 1 Apple
- ❖ 2 Kiwis
- ❖ 1 tablespoon flax seeds
- ❖ 1 tablespoon lucuma powder
- ❖ 1 cup crushed ice

Zucchini Apples Smoothie

- ❖ 1/2 cup zucchini
- ❖ 1 Apple
- ❖ 3/4 avocado
- ❖ 1 stalk Celery
- ❖ 1 Lemon
- ❖ 1 tbsp. Spirulina
- ❖ 1 1/2 cups crushed ice

Dandelion Smoothie

- ❖ 1 cup Dandelion greens
- ❖ 1 cup Spinach
- ❖ ½ cup tahini
- ❖ 1 Red Radish

* ❖ 1 tbsp. chia seeds
* ❖ 1 cup lavender tea

Broccoli Apple Smoothie

* ❖ 1 Apple
* ❖ 1 cup Broccoli
* ❖ 1 tbsp. Cilantro
* ❖ 1 Celery stalk
* ❖ 1 cup crushed ice
* ❖ 1 tbsp. crushed Seaweed

Salad Smoothie

* ❖ 1 cup Spinach
* ❖ ½ cucumber
* ❖ 1/2 small onion
* ❖ 2 tablespoons Parsley
* ❖ 2 tablespoons lemon juice
* ❖ 1 cup crushed ice
* ❖ 1 tbsp. olive oil or cumin oil
* ❖ ¼ cup Wheatgrass

SALAD DRESSINGS

Italian Dressing

Allergies: SF, GF, DF, EF, V, NF

- ❖ 2 tsp. olive oil or avocado oil
- ❖ lemon
- ❖ minced garlic
- ❖ salt

Yogurt Dressing

Allergies: SF, GF, DF, EF, V, NF

- ❖ 1 cup of plain low-fat Greek Yogurt or low-fat buttermilk
- ❖ 1 tsp. olive oil or avocado oil
- ❖ minced garlic
- ❖ salt
- ❖ lemon Occasionally, add a tsp. of mustard or some herbs like basil, oregano, marjoram, chives, thyme, parsley, dill, or mint.

If you like spicy hot food, add some cayenne to the Dressing. It will speed up your metabolism and have an interesting hot spicy effect in cold Yogurt or buttermilk.

SALADS

Large Fiber Loaded Salad with Italian Dressing

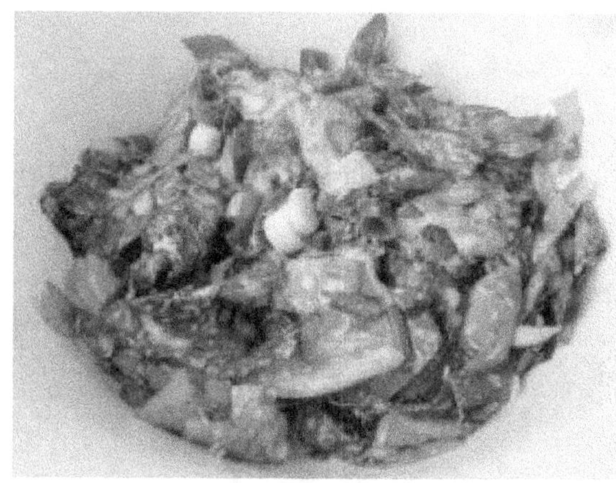

Allergies: SF, GF, EF, NF

- ❖ 2 cups of Spinach
- ❖ 1 cup of shredded cabbage, sauerkraut, or lettuce. Cabbage has more substance.
- ❖ Italian or Yogurt dressing
- ❖ Cayenne pepper (optional)
- ❖ Few sprigs of cilantro (optional)
- ❖ 2 spring (green) onions (optional)

Large Fiber Loaded Salad with Yogurt Dressing

Serves 1 - Allergies: SF, GF, EF, NF

- ❖ 2 cups of Spinach
- ❖ 1 cup of shredded cabbage or lettuce. Cabbage has more substance.
- ❖ Italian or Yogurt dressing

- ❖ Cayenne pepper (optional)
- ❖ Few sprigs of cilantro (optional)
- ❖ 2 spring (green) onions (optional

Large Fiber Loaded Salad as a meal on its own

Allergies: SF, GF, EF, NF

This is what I eat every second evening, and I can't get enough of it!!! This is the the real secret to lose weight while having a full stomach with grade A ingredients!!

- ❖ 2 cups of Spinach
- ❖ 2 cups of shredded cabbage
- ❖ Yogurt dressing
- ❖ Cayenne pepper (optional)
- ❖ Few sprigs of cilantro (optional)
- ❖ 3 spring (green) onions
- ❖ 10 o.z. low-fat farmers' cheese

- ● Pour yogurt dressing into the salad bowl.
- ● Add farmers' cheese and mix thoroughly.
- ● Cut spring onions in small pieces and add to the cheese mixture and mix.
- ● Add Spinach and cabbage and mix thoroughly.
- ● Add spices (optional).

Greek Salad

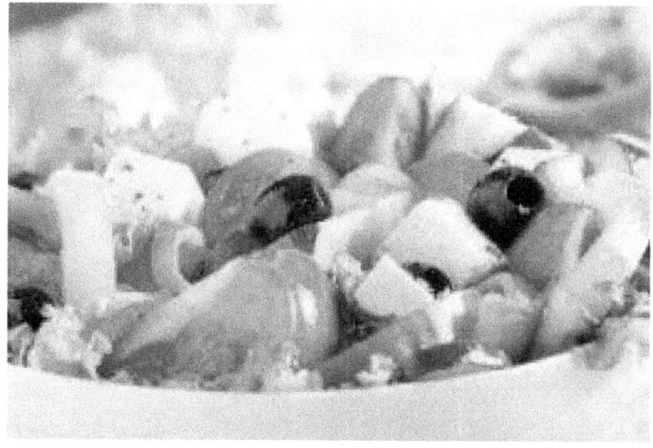

Allergies: SF, GF, EF, NF

- ❖ 1 head romaine lettuce
- ❖ 1/2 lb. plump tomatoes
- ❖ 3 oz. Greek or black olives, sliced
- ❖ 2 oz. sliced radishes
- ❖ 4 oz. low-fat feta or goat cheese
- ❖ 2 oz. anchovies (optional)

Dressing:

- ❖ 2 oz. olive oil or avocado oil
- ❖ 2 oz. fresh lemon juice
- ❖ 1/2 tsp. dried oregano
- ❖ 1/4 tsp. black pepper
- ❖ 1/4 tsp. salt
- ❖ 2 cloves garlic, minced

- ● Wash and cut lettuce into pieces. Slice tomatoes in quarters.
- ● Combine olives, lettuce, tomatoes, and radishes in a large bowl.
- ● Mix dressing ingredients and toss with vegetables.
- ● Pour out into a shallow serving bowl.
- ● Crumble feta/goat cheese overall, and arrange anchovy fillets on top (if desired).

Strawberry Spinach Salad

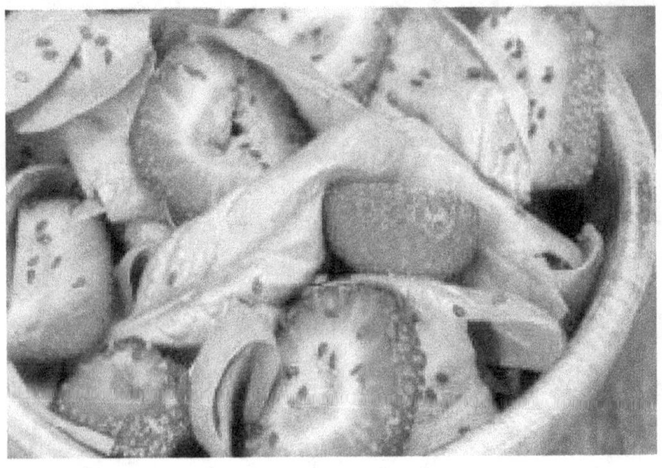

Allergies: SF, GF, DF, EF, V

Ingredients -

- ❖ 1 tbsp. black sesame seeds
- ❖ 1 tbsp. poppy seeds
- ❖ 1/4 cup olive oil or cumin oil
- ❖ 1/8 cup lemon juice
- ❖ 1/8 tsp. paprika
- ❖ 1/2 bag fresh spinach - chopped, washed, and dried
- ❖ 1 cup strawberries, sliced
- ❖ 1/4 cup toasted slivered almonds Instructions

- Whisk together the sesame seeds, olive oil, poppy seeds, paprika, lemon juice, and onion. Refrigerate.
- In a large bowl, combine the spinach, strawberries, and almonds.
- Pour dressing over salad.
- Toss and refrigerate 15 minutes before serving.

Cucumber, Cilantro, Quinoa Tabbouleh

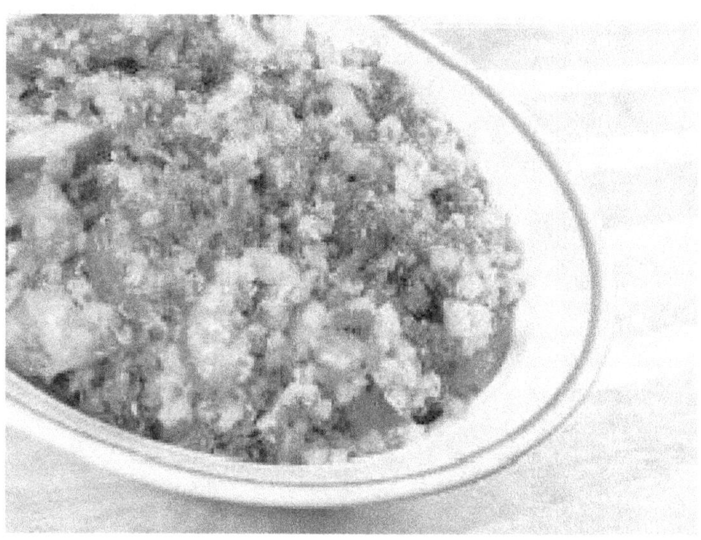

Serves 2

Allergies: SF, GF, DF, EF, NF, V

Ingredients -

- ❖ 1/2 cup cooked quinoa mixed with 1 tbsp. sesame seeds
- ❖ 1/2 cup chopped tomato and green pepper
- ❖ 1 cup chopped cucumber
- ❖ 1/2 cup chopped cilantro Dressing:
- ❖ 1 tbsp. olive oil or avocado oil
- ❖ 1 tbsp. fresh lemon juice
- ❖ pinch of black pepper
- ❖ pinch of sea salt

Instructions: Mix all ingredients.

Almond, Quinoa, Red Peppers & Arugula Salad

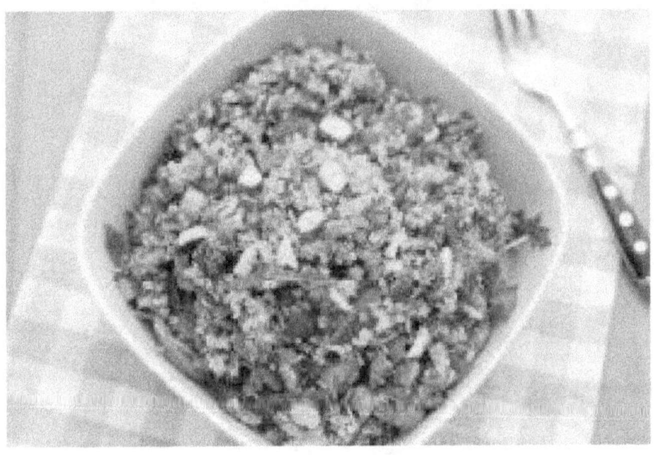

Serves 2

Allergies: SF, GF, DF, EF, NF, V

Ingredients -

- ❖ 1/2 cup cooked quinoa mixed with 1 tbsp. pumpkin seeds
- ❖ 1/2 cup chopped almonds
- ❖ 1 cup chopped arugula
- ❖ 1/2 cup sliced red peppers Dressing:
- ❖ 1 tbsp. olive oil or cumin oil
- ❖ 1 tbsp. fresh lemon juice
- ❖ pinch of black pepper
- ❖ pinch of sea salt

Instructions: Mix all ingredients.

Asparagus, Quinoa & Red Peppers Salad

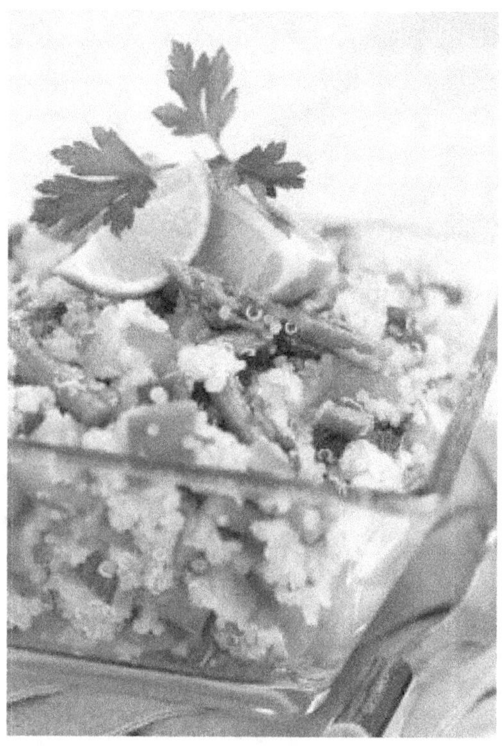

Serves 2

Allergies: SF, GF, DF, EF, NF, V

Ingredients –

- ❖ 1/2 cup cooked quinoa mixed with 1 tbsp. sunflower seeds
- ❖ 1 cup sliced red peppers
- ❖ 1 cup grilled asparagus
- ❖ Garnish with lime and parsley

Dressing:

- ❖ 1 tbsp. olive oil or avocado oil
- ❖ 1 tbsp. fresh lemon juice
- ❖ pinch of black pepper
- ❖ pinch of sea salt

Instructions: Mix all ingredients.

Chickpeas, Quinoa, Cucumber & Tomato Salad

Serves 2

Allergies: SF, GF, DF, EF, NF, V

Ingredients -

- ❖ 1/2 cup cooked quinoa mixed with 1 tbsp. sesame seeds
- ❖ 1/2 cup cooked chickpeas
- ❖ 1 cup chopped cucumber and green onions
- ❖ 1/2 cup chopped tomato Dressing:
- ❖ 1 tbsp. olive oil or avocado oil
- ❖ 1 tbsp. fresh lemon juice
- ❖ pinch of black pepper
- ❖ pinch of sea salt

Instructions: Mix all ingredients

Quinoa Salad

Allergies: SF, GF, EF

Ingredients -

For the salad

- ❖ 1/2 cup cooked quinoa
- ❖ 1/2 cup frozen green peas
- ❖ 1/4 cup low-fat feta cheese
- ❖ 4 oz. pork, cubed
- ❖ 1/8 cup freshly chopped basil and cilantro
- ❖ 1/8 cup almonds, pulsed in a food processor until crushed For the dressing
- ❖ 1/8 cup lemon juice (1 juicy lemon)
- ❖ 1/8 cup olive oil or cumin oil • 1/8 tsp. salt (more to taste)

Instructions

- ● Bring a pot of water to boil, and then lower the heat.

- Add the peas and cook covered until bright green. In the meantime, brown pork in a skillet.
- Toss the quinoa with the pork, peas, feta, herbs, and almonds.
- Puree all the dressing ingredients in the food processor.
- Toss the Dressing with the salad ingredients.
- Season generously with salt and pepper.
- Serve tossed with fresh baby spinach.

Cauliflower & Eggs Salad

Allergies: SF, GF, NF

Ingredients -

- 1 cup chopped Cauliflower
- 2 hardboiled eggs - chopped,
- 2 oz. shredded cheddar cheese, low-fat
- 1/2 red onion, celery,
- 1 dill pickles,
- 1 tbsp. Yellow mustard.

Mix all ingredients.

Greek Cucumber Salad

Allergies: SF, GF, EF, NF

Ingredients -

- 2 cucumbers, sliced
- 1 teaspoon salt
- 2 tbsp. lemon juice
- 1/4 tsp. paprika
- 1/4 tsp. white pepper
- 1/2 clove garlic, minced
- 2 fresh green onions, diced

❖ 1 cup thick Greek Yogurt

❖ 1/4 tsp. paprika

Instructions

● Slice cucumbers thinly sprinkle with salt and mix.

● Set aside for one hour.

● Mix lemon juice, Water, garlic, paprika, and white pepper, and set aside.

● Squeeze liquid from cucumber slices a few at a time, and place slices in the bowl.

● Discard liquid.

● Add lemon juice mixture, green onions, and Yogurt.

● Mix and sprinkle additional paprika or dill over the top. Chill for 1-2 hours

Mediterranean Salad

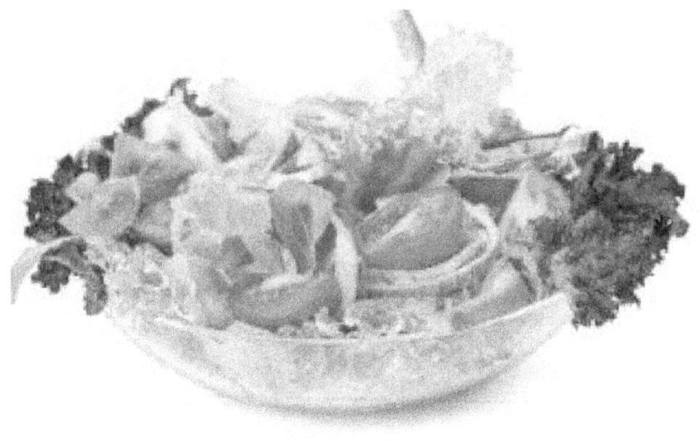

Allergies: SF, GF, DF, EF, V, NF

Ingredients -

❖ 1 small head romaine lettuce, torn

❖ 1 tomato, diced

❖ 1 small cucumber, sliced

❖ 1/2 green bell pepper, sliced

- ❖ 1/2 small onion, cut into rings
- ❖ 3 radishes, thinly sliced
- ❖ 1/4 cup flat-leaf parsley, chopped
- ❖ 1/4 cup olive oil or avocado oil
- ❖ 2 tbsp. lemon juice
- ❖ 1 garlic clove, minced
- ❖ Salt & pepper
- ❖ 1 tsp. fresh mint, minced

Instructions

- ● Combine lettuce, tomatoes, cucumber, pepper, onion, radishes & parsley in a salad bowl.
- ● Whisk together olive oil, lemon juice, Garlic, salt, pepper & mint.
- ● Pour over salad & toss to coat.

Apple Coleslaw

Allergies: SF, GF, DF, EF, V, NF

Ingredients -

- ❖ 2 cups chopped cabbage (various color)
- ❖ 1 tart apple chopped
- ❖ 1 celery, chopped
- ❖ 1 red pepper chopped
- ❖ 4 tsp. olive oil or avocado oil
- ❖ juice of 1 lemon
- ❖ 1 Tbs. lucuma powder (optional)
- ❖ dash sea salt

Instructions

- ● Toss the cabbage, apple, celery, and pepper together in a large bowl.
- ● In a smaller bowl, whisk the remaining ingredients.

● Drizzle over coleslaw and toss to coat.

Appetizers

Hummus

Allergies: SF, GF, DF, EF, V, NF

Ingredients -

- ❖ 1/2 cup cooked chickpeas (garbanzo beans)
- ❖ 1/2 small lemon
- ❖ 2 Tbsp. tahini
- ❖ Half of a garlic clove, minced
- ❖ 1 tbsp. olive oil or cumin oil, plus more for serving
- ❖ 1/2 tsp. salt
- ❖ 1/4 tsp. ground cumin
- ❖ 2 to 3 tbsp. water

❖ Dash of ground paprika for serving

Instructions

- Combine tahini and lemon juice and blend for 1 minute.
- Add the olive oil, minced garlic, cumin, and salt to the tahini and lemon mixture.
- Process for 30 seconds, scrape sides, and then process 30 seconds more.
- Add half of the chickpeas to the food processor and process for 1 minute.
- Scrape sides, add remaining chickpeas, and process for 1 to 2 minutes.
- Transfer the hummus into a bowl, then drizzle about 1 tbsp. of olive oil over the top and sprinkle with paprika.

Guacamole

Allergies: SF, GF, DF, EF, V, NF

Ingredients -

- ❖ 2 ripe avocados
- ❖ 2 tbsp. freshly squeezed lemon juice (1 lemon)
- ❖ 4 dashes hot pepper sauce
- ❖ 1/4 cup diced onion
- ❖ 1 garlic clove, minced
- ❖ 1/2 tsp. salt
- ❖ 1/2 tsp. ground black pepper
- ❖ 1 small tomato, seeded, and small-diced

Instructions

- Cut the avocados in half, remove the pits, and scoop the flesh out.
- Immediately add the lemon juice, hot pepper sauce, garlic, onion, salt, and pepper, and toss well.
- Dice avocados. Add the tomatoes.

- Mix well and taste for salt and pepper.

Baba Ghanoush

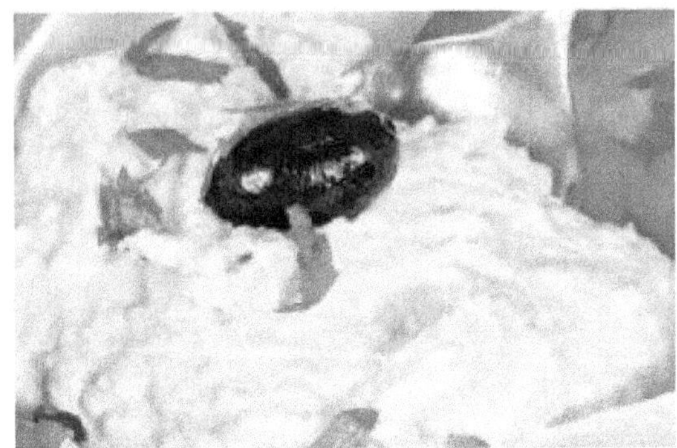

Allergies: SF, GF, DF, EF, V, NF

Ingredients -

- ❖ 1 eggplant
- ❖ 1/4 cup tahini, plus more as needed
- ❖ 1 garlic clove, minced
- ❖ 1/8 cup fresh lemon juice, plus more as needed
- ❖ 1 pinch ground cumin
- ❖ salt, to taste
- ❖ 1 tbsp. Extra-virgin olive oil or avocado oil
- ❖ 1 tbsp. chopped flat-leaf parsley
- ❖ 1/4 cup brine-cured black olives, such as Kalamata

Instructions:

- Grill eggplant for 10 to 15 minutes. Heat the oven (375 F).
- Put the eggplant on a baking sheet and bake 15-20 minutes or until very soft.
- Remove from the oven, let cool, and peel off and discard the skin.
- Put the eggplant flesh in a bowl. Using a fork, mash the eggplant to a paste.
- Add the 1/4 cup tahini, garlic, cumin, 1/4 cup lemon juice and mix well.
- Season with salt to taste.

● Transfer the mixture to a serving bowl and spread with the back of a spoon to form a shallow well.

● Drizzle the olive oil over the top and sprinkle with the parsley.

Espinacase la Catalana

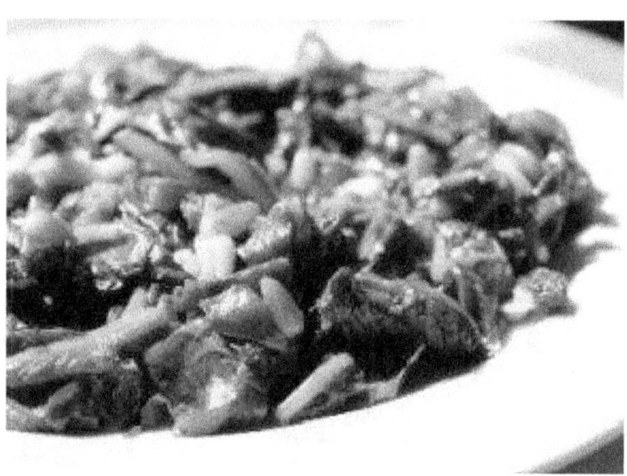

Allergies: SF, GF, DF, EF, V

- ❖ 1 cup Spinach
- ❖ 1 cloves garlic
- ❖ 2 tbsp cashews
- ❖ olive oil or avocado oil Instructions

Ingredients -

● Wash the Spinach and trim off the stems. Steam the Spinach for few minutes.

● Peel and slice the garlic.

● Pour a few tablespoons of olive oil and cover the bottom of a frying pan.

● Heat pan on medium and sauté garlic for 1-2 minutes.

● Add the cashews to the pan and continue to sauté for 1 minute.

● Add the Spinach and mix well, coating with oil.

● Salt to taste.

● Serve at room temperature.

Tapenade

Allergies: SF, GF, DF, EF, V, NF

Ingredients -

- ❖ 1/4 pound olives with pit removed
- ❖ 2 anchovy fillets, rinsed
- ❖ 1 small clove garlic, minced
- ❖ 2 tbsp. capers
- ❖ 2 fresh basil leaves
- ❖ 1 tbsp. freshly squeezed lemon juice
- ❖ 1 tbsp. extra-virgin olive oil or cumin oil

Instructions

- ● Rinse the olives in cold water.
- ● Place all ingredients in the bowl of a food processor.
- ● The process to combine until it becomes a coarse paste.
- ● Transfer to a bowl and serve.

SOUPS

Cream of Broccoli Soup

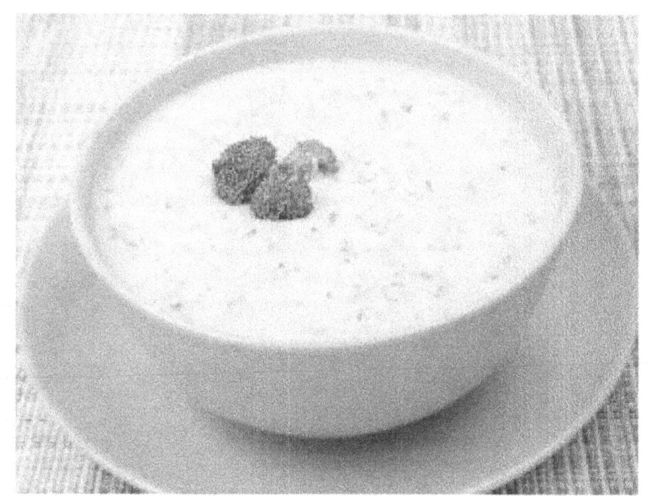

Allergies: SF, GF, EF, NF

Ingredients -

- ❖ 1 pound broccoli, fresh
- ❖ 1 cup of water
- ❖ 1/4 tsp. salt, pepper to taste
- ❖ 1/4 cup tapioca flour, mixed with 1 cup cold water
- ❖ 1/4 cup coconut cream
- ❖ 1/4 cup low-fat farmers' cheese Steam or boil Broccoli until it gets tender.

- ● Put 1 cup of water and coconut cream on top of a double boiler.
- ● Add salt, cheese, and pepper.
- ● Heat until cheese gets melted.
- ● Add Broccoli. Mix water and tapioca flour in a small bowl.
- ● Stir tapioca mixture into cheese mixture in double boiler and heat until soup thickens.

Lentil Soup

Allergies: SF, GF, DF, EF, NF

Ingredients -

- ❖ 1 tbsp. olive oil or avocado oil
- ❖ 1/2 cup finely chopped onion
- ❖ 1/4 cup chopped carrot
- ❖ 1/4 cup chopped celery
- ❖ 1 teaspoons salt
- ❖ 1/2 pound lentils
- ❖ 1/2 cup chopped tomatoes
- ❖ 1-quart chicken or vegetable broth
- ❖ 1/4 tsp. ground coriander & toasted cumin

Instructions

- ● Place the olive oil into a large Dutch oven.
- ● Set over medium heat.

- Once hot, add the celery, onion, carrot, and salt and do until the onions are translucent.
- Add the lentils, tomatoes, cumin, broth, and coriander and stir to combine.
- Increase the heat and bring just to a boil.
- Reduce the heat, cover, and simmer at a low until the lentils are tender (approx. 35 to 40 minutes).
- Puree with a bender to your preferred consistency (optional). Serve immediately.

Bouillabaisse

Allergies: SF, GF, DF, EF, NF

Ingredients -

- 1 pound of 3 different kinds of fish fillets
- 1/4 cup Coconut oil
- 1 pound of Oysters, clams, or mussels
- 1/3 cup cooked shrimp, crab, or lobster meat, or rock lobster tails
- 1/3 cup thinly sliced onions
- 1 Shallot or the white parts of 1 leek, thinly sliced
- 1 clove garlic, crushed
- 1 small tomato, chopped
- 1/2 sweet red pepper, chopped
- 2 stalks celery, thinly sliced
- 1-inch slice of fennel or 1/2 tsp. of fennel seed
- 1 sprigs fresh thyme or 1/4 tsp. dried thyme
- 1 bay leaf
- 1 whole cloves
- Zest of half an orange
- 1/4 tsp. saffron
- 1 teaspoons salt
- 1/4 tsp. ground black pepper
- 1/3 cup clam juice or fish broth
- 1 Tbps lemon juice

❖ 1/3 cup white wine

Instructions

- In a large saucepan, heat 1/8 cup of the coconut oil.
- When it is hot, add onions and shallots (or leeks). Sauté for a minute.
- Add crushed garlic and sweet red pepper.
- Add celery, tomato, and fennel.
- Stir the vegetables until well coated.
- Add another 1/8 cup of coconut oil, bay leaf, thyme, cloves, and the orange zest.
- Cook until the onion is golden.
- Cut fish fillets into 2-inch pieces.
- Add 1 cup of water and the pieces of fish to the vegetable mixture.
- Bring to a boil, reduce heat, and let it simmer, uncovered, for about 10 minutes.
- Add clams, oysters, or mussels (optional) and crabmeat, shrimp, or lobster tails, cut into pieces.
- Add salt, saffron, and pepper.
- Add lemon juice, clam juice, and white wine.
- Bring to a simmer again and cook for 5 minutes longer.

Gaspacho

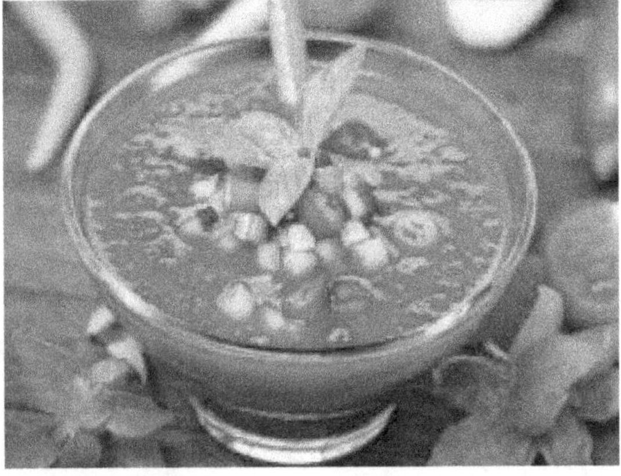

Allergies: SF, GF, DF, EF, V, NF

Ingredients -

- ❖ 1/4 cup of flax seeds meal
- ❖ 1 pound tomatoes, diced
- ❖ 1 red pepper or one green pepper, diced
- ❖ 1 small cucumber, peeled and diced
- ❖ 1 cloves of garlic, peeled and crushed
- ❖ ¼ cup extra virgin olive oil or cumin oil
- ❖ 1 tbsp. lemon juice
- ❖ Salt, to taste

Instructions

- Mix the peppers, tomatoes, and cucumber with the crushed garlic and olive oil in a blender bowl. Add flax meal to the mixture.
- Blend until smooth.
- Add salt and lemon juice to taste and stir well.
- Refrigerate. Serve with black olives, hardboiled egg, cilantro, mint or parsley.

Italian Beef Soup

Allergies: SF, GF, DF, EF, NF

Ingredients -

- ❖ 1/3 pound minced beef
- ❖ 1 clove garlic, minced
- ❖ 1 cups beef broth
- ❖ 1 large tomato
- ❖ 1/2 cup sliced carrots
- ❖ 1/2 cup cooked beans
- ❖ 1 small zucchini, cubed

- ❖ 1 cups Spinach - rinsed and torn
- ❖ 1/8 tsp. black pepper
- ❖ 1/8 tsp. Salt Brown Beef with Garlic in a stockpot.

- Stir in broth, carrots, and tomatoes.
- Season with salt and pepper.
- Reduce heat, cover, and simmer for 15 minutes.
- Stir in beans with liquid and zucchini. Cover, and simmer until zucchini is tender.
- Remove from heat, add Spinach, and cover.
- Serve after 5 minutes.

Black Bean Soup

Allergies: SF, GF, DF, EF, NF

Ingredients -

- ❖ 1 Tbsp. cup Coconut Oil
- ❖ 1/4 cup Onion, Diced
- ❖ 1/4 cup Carrots, Diced
- ❖ 1/4 cup Green Bell Pepper, Diced
- ❖ 1 cup beef broth
- ❖ 1 pound cooked Black Beans
- ❖ 1 tbsp. lemon juice
- ❖ 1 teaspoons chopped garlic
- ❖ 1 teaspoons Salt
- ❖ 1/4 tsp. Black Pepper, Ground
- ❖ 1 teaspoons Chili Powder
- ❖ 4 oz. pork
- ❖ 1 tbsp. tapioca flour
- ❖ 2 tbsp. Water

Instructions

- Place coconut oil, onion, carrot, and bell pepper in a stockpot.
- Cook the veggies until tender.
- Bring broth to a boil.
- Add cooked beans, broth, and the remaining ingredients (except tapioca flour and 2 tbsp. water) to the vegetables.
- Bring that mixture to a simmer and cook for approximately 15 minutes.
- Puree 1 quart of the soup in a blender and put back into the pot.
- Combine the tapioca flour and 2 tbsp. Water in a separate bowl.
- Add the tapioca flour mixture to the bean soup and bring to a boil for 1 minute.

GRILLED MEATS & SALAD

Chicken and Large Fiber Loaded Salad with Italian Dressing

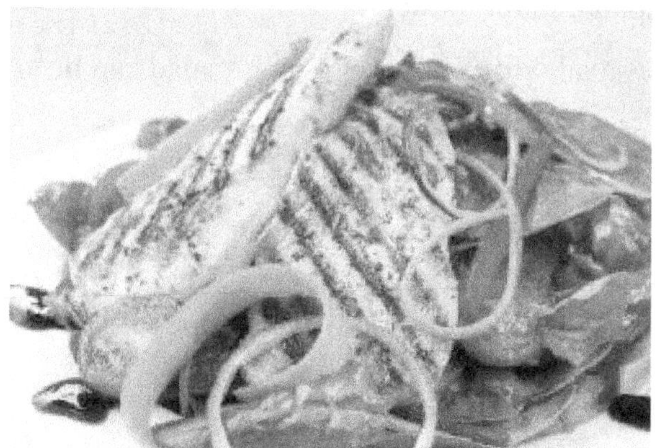

Allergies: SF, GF, EF, NF

- 2 6oz. pieces of ChickenChicken (or turkey), skinless, boneless grilled, or prepared in the skillet.

- Large mixed Spinach and lettuce salad with Italian Dressing and half a tsp of mustard. Salad can be as large as you want, but use half a cup of the Dressing.

Salmon with Large Fiber Loaded Salad with Italian Dressing

Allergies: SF, GF, DF, EF, NF

- 2 Salmon steaks grilled or prepared in the skillet.
- Large mixed Spinach and lettuce salad with "Italian Dressing" and some thyme sprinkled on top of it. Salad can be as large as you want, but use the prescribed amount of the Dressing.

Ground Beef Patty with Large Fiber Loaded Salad with Yogurt Dressing

Allergies: SF, GF, EF, NF

- 2 5oz. Lean ground beef patty grilled or prepared in the skillet.
- Large mixed Spinach and shredded cabbage salad with Yogurt Dressing. Salad can be as large as you want, but use half a cup of a dressing

STEWS, CHILIES, AND CURRIES

Vegetarian Chili

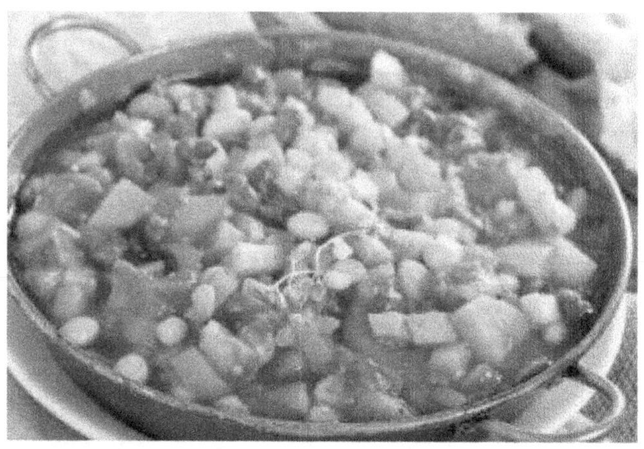

Allergies: SF, GF, DF, EF, V, NF

Ingredients -

- ❖ 1 tbsp. coconut oil
- ❖ 1/2 cup chopped onions
- ❖ 1/2 cup chopped carrots
- ❖ 1 cloves garlic, minced
- ❖ 1/2 cup chopped green bell pepper
- ❖ 1/2 cup chopped red bell pepper
- ❖ 1/4 cup chopped celery
- ❖ 1/2 tbsp. chili powder
- ❖ 1/2 cups chopped mushrooms
- ❖ 1 cup chopped tomatoes
- ❖ 1 cups cooked kidney beans
- ❖ 1/2 tbsp. ground cumin
- ❖ 1/2 teaspoons oregano
- ❖ 1/2 teaspoons crushed basil leaves

Instructions

- Heat coconut oil in a large saucepan and add onions, carrots, and garlic; sauté until tender.
- Stir in green pepper, red pepper, celery, and chili powder.
- Cook, often stirring, until vegetables are tender, about 6 minutes.
- To the vegetables, add mushrooms; cook 4 minutes. Stir in tomatoes, kidney beans, corn, cumin, oregano, and basil.
- Bring to a boil.
- Reduce heat to medium. Cover and simmer for 20 minutes, stirring occasionally.

Braised Green Peas with Beef

Allergies: SF, GF, DF, EF, NF

Ingredients -

- ❖ 2 cups fresh or frozen green peas
- ❖ 1 onion, finely chopped

- ❖ 2 cloves of garlic, thinly sliced and 1/2 inch of peeled/sliced fresh ginger (if you like)
- ❖ 1/2 tsp. red pepper flakes, or to taste
- ❖ 1 tomato, roughly chopped
- ❖ 2 chopped carrots
- ❖ 2 tbsp. coconut oil
- ❖ 1 cup chicken broth
- ❖ 10 oz. cubed Beef
- ❖ Salt and freshly ground black pepper

- ● Heat the coconut oil in a skillet over medium heat. Sauté the onion, garlic, and ginger until they are soft
- ● . Add the red pepper, carrot, and tomatoes and sauté until the tomato begins to soften.
- ● Add in the green peas.
- ● Add cubed Lean Beef.
- ● Add in the broth and simmer over medium heat. Cover and cook until the peas are tender.
- ● Season to taste with salt and pepper.

White Chicken Chili

Allergies: SF, GF, DF, EF, NF

Ingredients -

- ❖ 2 large boneless, skinless chicken breasts
- ❖ 1 green bell peppers
- ❖ 1/2 yellow onion
- ❖ 1/2 jalapeno
- ❖ 1/4 cup diced green chilies (optional)
- ❖ 1/4 cup of spring onions
- ❖ 1 tbsp. coconut oil
- ❖ 1/2 cup cooked white beans
- ❖ 2 cups chicken or vegetable broth
- ❖ 1/2 tsp. ground cumin

❖ 1/8 tsp. cayenne pepper

❖ salt to taste

Instructions

- Bring a pot of water to boil.

- Add the chicken breasts and cook until cooked through.

- Drain water and allow ChickenChicken to cool. When cold, shred and set aside.

- Dice the bell peppers, jalapeno, and onion.

- Melt the coconut oil in a pot over high heat.

- Add the peppers and onions and sauté until soft, approx. 8-10 minutes.

- Add the broth, beans, ChickenChicken, and spices to the pot.

- Stir and bring to a low boil. Cover and simmer for 25-30 minutes.

- Simmer for 10 more minutes and stir occasionally. Remove from heat.

- Let stand for 10 minutes to thicken. Top with cilantro.

Kale Pork

Allergies: SF, GF, DF, EF, NF

Ingredients -

❖ 1 tbsp. coconut oil

❖ 1/2 pound pork tenderloin, trimmed and cut into 1-inch pieces • 1/4 tsp. salt

❖ 1/2 medium onion, finely chopped

❖ 2 cloves garlic, minced

❖ 1 teaspoons paprika

❖ 1/8 tsp. crushed red pepper (optional) • 1/2 cup white wine

❖ 2 plump tomatoes, chopped

❖ 2 cups chicken broth

❖ 1/2 bunch kale, chopped

❖ 1 cups cooked white beans

Instructions

- Heat oil in a pot over medium heat.

- Add pork, season with salt, and cook until no longer pink.

- Transfer to a plate and leave juices in the pot.

- Add onion to the pot and cook until it turns translucent

- . Add paprika, garlic, and crushed red pepper and cook for about 30 seconds.

- Add tomatoes and wine, increase heat and stir to scrape up any browned bits.

- Add broth. Bring to a boil.

- Add KaleKale and stir until it wilts.

- Lower the heat and simmer until the KaleKale is tender.

- Stir in beans, pork, and pork juices.

- Simmer for 2 more minutes.

STIR-FRIES

Pork and Bok Choy / Celery Stir Fry

Allergies: SF, GF, DF, EF, NF

10 oz. Lean Pork Tenderloin and 2 cups Bok Choy / Celery stir fry.

- Use as many veggies as you want, or replace Bok Choy with Kale. Season with fish sauce.

Lemon Chicken Stir Fry

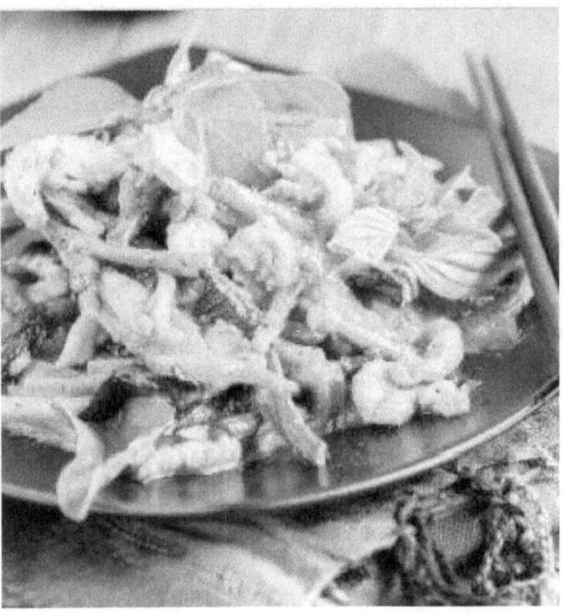

Allergies: SF, GF, DF, EF, NF

Ingredients -

- ❖ 1/2 lemon
- ❖ 1/4 cup chicken broth
- ❖ 1 tbsp. fish sauce
- ❖ 1 teaspoons arrowroot flour
- ❖ 1/2 tbsp. coconut oil
- ❖ 1/2 pound boneless, skinless chicken breasts, trimmed and cut into 1-inch pieces
- ❖ 5 ounces mushrooms, halved or quartered
- ❖ 1 cup snow peas, stems and strings removed
- ❖ 1 bunch scallions, cut into 1-inch pieces, white and green parts divided
- ❖ 1 tbsp. chopped garlic

Instructions

- ● Grate 1 tsp. Lemon zest. Juice the lemon and mix 3 tbsp. Of the juice with broth, fish sauce, and arrowroot flour in a small bowl.
- ● Heat oil in a skillet over high heat.
- ● Add ChickenChicken and cook, occasionally stirring, until just cooked through.
- ● Transfer to a plate.
- ● Add mushrooms to the pan and cook until the mushrooms are tender.
- ● Add snow peas, garlic, scallion whites, and the lemon zest.

- Cook, stirring, around 30 seconds.
- Add the broth to the pan and cook, stirring, 2 to 3 minutes.
- Add scallion greens and the ChickenChicken and any accumulated juices and stir.

Pan-seared Brussels sprouts

Serves 2

Allergies: SF, GF, DF, EF, NF

Ingredients -

- ❖ 6 oz. cubed pork
- ❖ 2 tbsp. coconut oil
- ❖ 1 pound Brussels sprouts, halved
- ❖ 1/2 large onion, chopped
- ❖ Salt and ground black pepper

Instructions

- Cook pork in a skillet over high heat.
- Remove to a plate and chop.
- In the same pan with pork fat, add coconut oil over high heat.
- Add onions and Brussels sprouts and cook, occasionally stirring, until sprouts are golden brown.
- Season with salt and pepper to taste, and put the pork back into the pan.
- Serve immediately

Beef and Broccoli Stir Fry

Allergies: SF, GF, DF, EF, NF

- ❖ 10 oz. of lean Beef and 2 cups broccoli stir fry.

- Use as much Broccoli as you want or replace Broccoli with Kale.

MEATS

Baked Chicken Breast with Fresh Basil

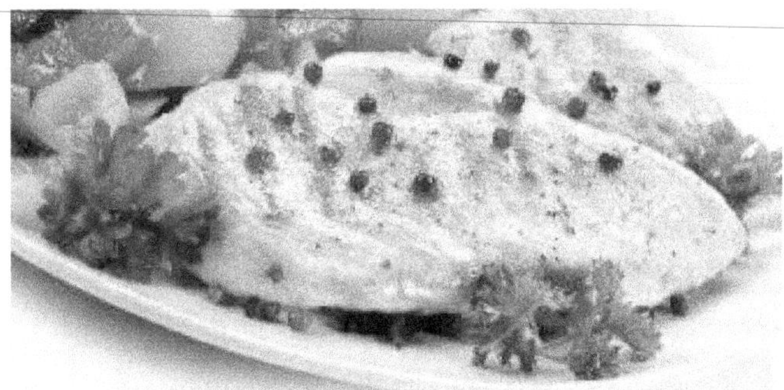

Allergies: SF, GF, EF, NF

Ingredients -

- ❖ 2 boneless skinless chicken breast

- ❖ 1/4 cup low-fat Yogurt
- ❖ 1/4 cup chopped basil
- ❖ 1 tsp. arrowroot flour
- ❖ 2 Tbsp. oatmeal, coarsely ground

Instructions

- Arrange ChickenChicken in a baking dish. Combine basil, Yogurt, and arrowroot flour;
- mix well and spread over ChickenChicken.
- Mix oatmeal with salt and pepper to taste and sprinkle over ChickenChicken.
- Bake chicken at 375 degrees in the oven for half an hour.

Roast Chicken with Rosemary

Allergies: SF, GF, DF, EF, NF

- ❖ 2 chicken pieces, skinned
- ❖ salt and pepper to taste
- ❖ 1 onion, quartered
- ❖ 2 Tbsp. chopped rosemary

Instructions -

- Heat the oven to 350F.
- Sprinkle meat with salt and pepper.
- Cover with the onion and rosemary.
- Place in a baking dish and bake in the preheated oven until ChickenChicken is cooked through.

Carne Asada

Allergies: SF, GF, DF, EF, NF

Marinade:

- ❖ Mix the garlic, jalapeno, cilantro, salt, and pepper to make a paste.
- ❖ Put the paste in a container.
- ❖ Add the oil and lime juice.
- ❖ Shake it up to combine.
- ❖ Use as a marinade for Beef or as a table condiment.

Instructions

- Put the 1 pound flank steak in a baking dish and pour the marinade over it.
- Refrigerate up to 8 hours.
- Take the steak out of the marinade and season it on both sides with salt and pepper.
- Grill (or broil) the steak for 7 to 10 minutes per side, turning once, until medium-rare.
- Put the steak on a cutting board and allow the juices to settle (5 minutes).
- Thinly slice the steak across the grain.

CASSEROLES

Broccoli Chicken Casserole

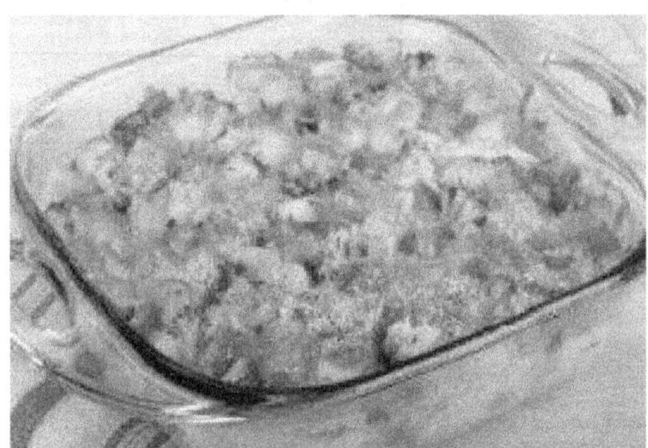

Allergies: SF, GF, NF

Ingredients -

- ❖ 2 cups broccoli florets
- ❖ 10 oz. skinless, boneless chicken (or turkey) pieces (breast or dark meat)
- ❖ 2 tsp of flax seeds meal
- ❖ Salt, pepper
- ❖ 2 eggs - beaten
- ❖ 1 cup of Yogurt Dressing (or coconut milk, if you don't like the sourish tang)
- ❖ 1/2 cup of chicken broth
- ❖ 4 tbsp. Of grated low-fat cheddar cheese,

- ● Heat the oven to 400°. Cook broccoli for around 5 minutes.
- ● Take Broccoli out and add ChickenChicken (or turkey) and simmer for 15 minutes.
- ● Cut ChickenChicken (or turkey) into cubes and add it to the Broccoli.
- ● Combine broth, flax, salt, and pepper in a pan and mix.
- ● Bring to a boil over high heat and cook for 1 minute, stirring constantly. Remove from heat.
- ● Add yogurt dressing, beaten egg, and then half of the cheese, stirring until well combined.
- ● Add sauce to broccoli mixture, and stir gently until combined.
- ● Put the mixture in a small casserole dish oiled with some coconut oil.
- ● Put remaining cheese on top, sprinkle.
- ● Bake at 400° for 50 minutes or until mixture bubbles at the edges and cheese begins to brown.
- ● Remove from oven and let cool for 5 minutes.

Beef Meatballs Broccoli Casserole

Allergies: SF, GF

Ingredients -

- ❖ 2 cups broccoli florets

- ❖ 10 oz. beef meatballs (see separate recipe)
- ❖ 2 tsp of almond flour
- ❖ Salt, pepper
- ❖ 2 eggs - beaten
- ❖ 1 cup of Yogurt Dressing
- ❖ 1/2 cup of chicken broth
- ❖ 2 tbsp. of grated low-fat cheddar cheese

Instructions

- ● Heat oven to 400F. Cook broccoli for around 5 minutes.
- ● Prepare beef meatballs as in the recipe above.
- ● Combine broth, flour, salt, and pepper in a saucepan, stirring with a whisk until smooth.
- ● Bring to a boil over medium-high heat; cook 1 minute, stirring constantly.
- ● Remove from heat.
- ● Add yogurt dressing, beaten egg, and then half of the cheese, stirring until well combined.
- ● Add sauce to broccoli mixture, and stir gently until combined.
- ● Put the mixture in a small casserole dish oiled with some coconut oil.
- ● Sprinkle with remaining cheese.
- ● Bake at 400° for 50 minutes or until mixture bubbles at the edges and cheese begins to brown.
- ● Remove from oven and let cool for 5 minutes.
- ● Serve with large Fiber Loaded Salad with Italian Dressing.

Beef Meatballs Cauliflower Casserole

Allergies: SF, GF

Ingredients -

- ❖ 2 cups cauliflower florets

- ❖ 10 oz. beef meatballs (see separate recipe)
- ❖ 2 tsp of almond flour
- ❖ Salt, pepper
- ❖ 2 eggs - beaten
- ❖ 1 cup of Yogurt Dressing
- ❖ 1/2 cup of chicken broth
- ❖ 2 tbsp of grated low-fat cheddar cheese

Instructions

- Heat oven to 400°.
- Cook cauliflower for around 5 minutes.
- Prepare beef meatballs as in the recipe above. Combine soup, flour, salt, and pepper in a saucepan, stirring with a whisk until smooth. Bring to a boil over medium-high heat; cook 1 minute, stirring constantly.
- Remove from heat.
- Add yogurt dressing, beaten egg, and then half of the cheese, stirring until well combined.
- Add sauce to the cauliflower mixture, and stir gently until combined.
- Put the mixture in a small casserole dish oiled with some coconut oil. Sprinkle with remaining cheese.
- Bake at 400° for 50 minutes or until mixture bubbles at the edges and cheese begins to brown. Remove from oven and let cool for 5 minutes.
- Serve with large Fiber Loaded Salad with Italian Dressing.

"BREADED" "FRIED" FOOD

Breaded Tilapia

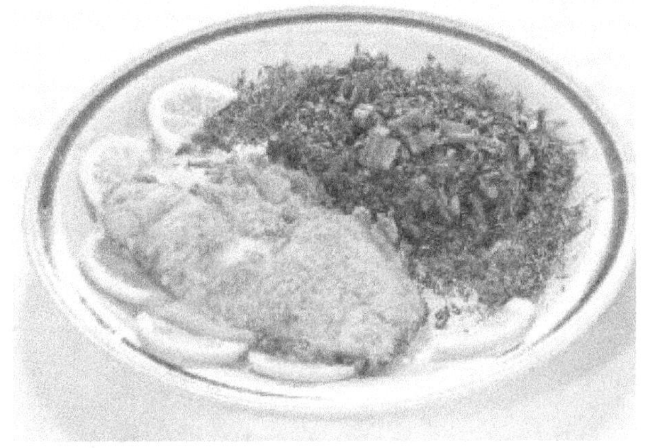

Allergies: SF, GF, DF, NF

Ingredients -

- ❖ 1/2 cup coconut meal for breading
- ❖ 1/4 tsp. pepper
- ❖ 1/4 tsp. minced garlic
- ❖ 1/4 tsp. paprika
- ❖ 1/8 tsp. salt
- ❖ 1 large egg whites (or whole eggs), beaten
- ❖ 1/2 pound tilapia fillets, cut into 1/2-by-3-inch strips

Instructions

- Heat oven to 400°F. Set a wire rack on a baking sheet and coat with some coconut oil.
- Place coconut, pepper, Garlic, paprika, and salt in a blender and process until finely.
- Transfer to a shallow dish.
- Place egg whites in a second dish. Dip every piece of fish in the egg and then coat all sides with the coconut breading mixture.
- Place on the prepared rack.
- Sprinkle some drops of olive oil over each piece.
- Bake until the fish is cooked through. Breading should be golden brown.
- Serve with large FiberFiber loaded salad.

Breaded Chicken

Allergies: SF, GF, DF, NF

Ingredients -

- ❖ 1/2 cup flax seeds meal for breading
- ❖ 1/4 tsp. pepper
- ❖ 1/4 tsp. minced garlic
- ❖ 1/4 tsp. paprika

- ❖ 1/8 tsp. salt
- ❖ 1 large egg whites (or whole eggs), beaten
- ❖ 1/2 pound skinless, boneless chicken pieces

Instructions

- Heat oven to 400°F. Set a wire rack on a baking sheet; coat with some coconut oil.
- Place flax, pepper, Garlic, paprika, and salt in a food processor or blender and process until finely.
- Transfer to a shallow dish.
- Place egg whites in a second dish. Dip every piece of ChickenChicken in the egg and then coat all sides with the flax breading mixture.
- Place on the prepared rack.
- Sprinkle some drops of olive oil over each piece.
- Bake until the ChickenChicken is cooked through, and the breading is golden brown and crisp, about 8 minutes each side.
- Serve with a large FiberFiber loaded salad.

Lemon Pork with Asparagus

Allergies: SF, GF, DF, EF, NF

Ingredients -

- ❖ 1/2 lb. pork chops
- ❖ 2 Tbsp. buckwheat flour
- ❖ 1/4 tsp. salt
- ❖ 1 tbsp. coconut oil
- ❖ Pepper
- ❖ 1/2 cup chopped asparagus
- ❖ 1 lemons, sliced

Instructions

- Place the flour and salt in a dish and gently toss each chop in the dish to coat. Melt the coconut oil in a large skillet over medium-high heat.
- Add the ChickenChicken and sauté until golden brown on each side.
- Sprinkle each side with the pepper directly in the pan.
- When the chops are cooked through, transfer them to a plate.
- Add the lemon slices and asparagus to the pan.
- When the asparagus and the lemons are done, add the chops back to the pan.

PIZZA

Meat Pizza

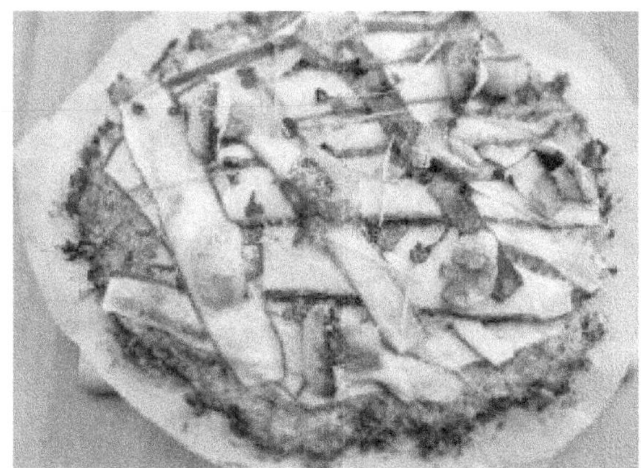

Allergies: SF, GF, EF, NF

Ingredients -

- ❖ 1/2 cup cooked and minced chicken breast
- ❖ 1/2 cup low-fat cheddar, shredded
- ❖ 1/2 tbsp. minced onion & few basil leaves
- ❖ 1/2 tsp garlic minced

Instructions

- Preheat oven to 425 degrees Fahrenheit. Process chicken, onion, and garlic together.
- The mixture will be a dense crumb consistency.
- Press chicken mixture on parchment paper on a cookie sheet. Bake for 12 minutes. Let cool for five minutes.
- Top with 1/4 cup of tomato sauce, a handful of low-fat cheese, basil, and mushrooms (shiitake). Bake for 6-8 minutes more, or until toppings are melted.
- Let cool for five minutes. Slice and serve. Alternatively, you may want to try the cauliflower crust version:
- Grate half of the large Cauliflower and steam it for 15 minutes.
- Squeeze the excess water out and let cool. Mix in 2 eggs, one cup low-fat mozzarella, and salt and pepper.
- Pat into a 10-inch round on the prepared cookie sheet.
- Brush with oil and bake until golden. Add the topping as above.

SIDE DISHES

Roasted curried Cauliflower

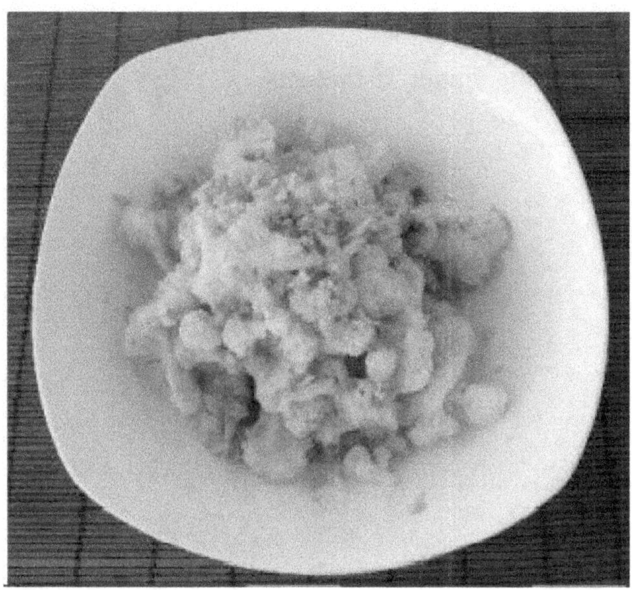

Allergies: SF, GF, DF, EF, NF

Ingredients -

- ❖ 2 cups cauliflower florets
- ❖ 1/2 chopped small onion
- ❖ 1/4 tsp. coriander seeds
- ❖ 1/4 tsp. cumin seeds
- ❖ 2 Tbsp. cup olive oil or cumin oil
- ❖ 1/4 cup lemon juice
- ❖ 1 teaspoon curry paste
- ❖ 1/4 tbsp. hot paprika
- ❖ 1/4 teaspoons salt
- ❖ 2 tbsp. cup chopped cilantro

Instructions

- Heat oven to 450°F. Place cauliflower florets in a large roasting pan.
- Add onions to Cauliflower.
- Dry toast coriander and cumin seeds in a skillet over medium heat until slightly browned, about 5 minutes.
- Crush in a mortar with pestle.
- Place seeds in a bowl. Whisk in oil, lemon juice, curry paste, paprika, and salt.
- Pour Dressing over vegetables and toss to coat.

- Spread vegetables in a single layer and sprinkle with pepper.
- Roast vegetables until tender, occasionally stirring, about 35 minutes.
- Sprinkle cilantro and serve warm.

Roasted Cauliflower with Tahini sauce

Allergies: SF, GF, DF, EF, V, NF

Ingredients -

- 2 Tbsp. cup extra-virgin olive oil or avocado oil
- 1 tsp. ground cumin
- 1 smaller cauliflower head, cored and cut into 1 1/2" florets
- Salt and ground black pepper
- 1/4 cup tahini
- 1 cloves garlic, smashed and minced into a paste
- Juice of 1/4 lemon

Instructions

- Roast Cauliflower like in the previous recipe.
- Meanwhile, combine tahini, lemon juice, garlic, and 1/4 cup water in a bowl and season with salt. Serve Cauliflower hot or at room temperature with tahini sauce.

Asparagus with mushrooms and hazelnuts

Ingredients - Allergies: SF, GF, DF, EF, V

- 1 tbsp. lemon juice
- 1/8 tsp sea salt

- ❖ Ground black pepper, to taste
- ❖ 1/2 pound fresh asparagus, ends trimmed
- ❖ 1 tbsp. coconut oil
- ❖ 2 cups mushrooms
- ❖ 1/4 cup green onions, sliced
- ❖ 1 tbsp. hazelnuts, toasted and finely chopped

Instructions

- Add the lemon juice, 1/2 tbsp. Of the oil, salt, and pepper in a small bowl
- . Boil water in a pan and add the asparagus.
- Boil for few minutes.
- Heat the remaining 1/2 tbsp.
- Oil in a pan on high heat.
- Add mushrooms and cook them until they are soft.
- Add green onions and sauté one more minute.
- Add the asparagus, and cook for another 3 minutes.
- Remove from the heat and slowly add in the lemon juice mixture.
- Add the toasted hazelnuts over the top.

Chard and Cashew Sauté

Serves 2

Allergies: SF, GF, DF, EF, V, NF

Ingredients -

- ❖ 1 bunch Swiss chard
- ❖ 1/2 cup cashews
- ❖ 1 tbsp. coconut oil
- ❖ Sea salt (optional)

❖ ground black pepper

Instructions

- Wash Swiss chard and remove tough stems.
- Heat a skillet over medium heat, and add oil when hot.
- Chop Swiss chard into thin strips.
- Add Swiss chard to the hot skillet, along with cashews.
- Sauté only 1 minute.
- Season with sea salt and ground black pepper to taste and serve warm.

Cauliflower rice side dish

Serves 2

Allergies: SF, GF, DF, EF, V, NF

Ingredients -

- ❖ 1 head Cauliflower
- ❖ 2 Tbs coconut oil
- ❖ Sea salt, garlic, ginger, or ground black pepper (optional seasonings)

Instructions

- Place the cauliflower into a food processor and pulse it until a grainy rice-like consistency.
- Season with sea salt and ground black pepper.
- Meanwhile, heat a large pan over medium heat.
- Add coconut oil when hot.
- Sauté Cauliflower in a pan with oil and any additional seasonings if desired.

CROCKPOT

Slow Cooker Pepper Steak

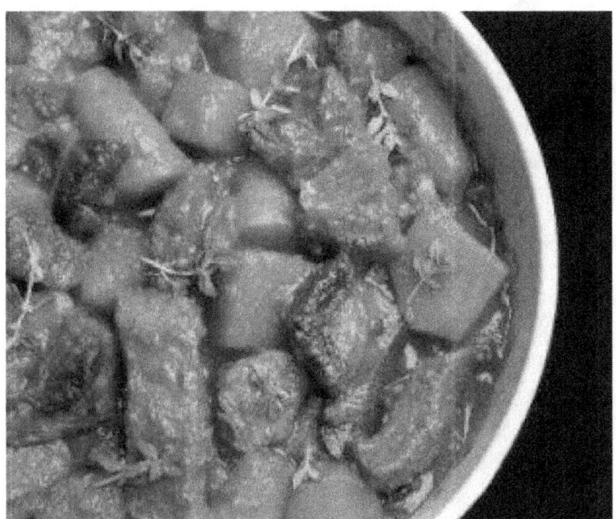

Allergies: SF, GF, DF, EF, NF

Ingredients -

- ❖ 1 pounds beef sirloin, cut into 2-inch strips
- ❖ 1/2 tbsp. minced garlic
- ❖ 1 tbsp. coconut oil
- ❖ 1/2 cup Beef Broth
- ❖ 1/2 tbsp. tapioca flour
- ❖ 1/4 cup chopped onion
- ❖ 1 cup carrots
- ❖ 1/2 cup chopped tomatoes
- ❖ 1/2 tsp. salt

Instructions

- Sprinkle Beef with Minced Garlic.
- Heat the coconut oil in a skillet and brown the seasoned beef sirloin strips.
- Transfer to a slow cooker.
- Mix in tapioca flour in broth until dissolved.
- Pour broth into the slow cooker with meat.
- Add carrots, onion, chopped tomatoes, and salt.
- Cover and cook on high for 3 to 4 hours, or on Low for 6 to 8 hours.

Pork Tenderloin with peppers and onions

Allergies: SF, GF, DF, EF, NF

Ingredients -

- ❖ 1 tbsp. coconut oil
- ❖ 3/4 pound pork loin
- ❖ 1/2 tbsp. caraway seeds
- ❖ 1/4 tsp sea salt
- ❖ 1/8 tsp ground black pepper
- ❖ 1/2 red onion, thinly sliced
- ❖ 1 red bell peppers, sliced
- ❖ 2 cloves of garlic, minced
- ❖ 1/4 cup chicken broth

Instructions

- Wash and chop vegetables. Slice pork loin, and season with black pepper, caraway seeds, and sea salt.
- Heat a pan over medium heat.
- Add coconut oil when hot.
- Add pork loin and brown slightly.
- Add onions and mushrooms, and continue to sauté until onions are translucent.
- Add peppers, garlic, and chicken broth.
- Simmer until vegetables are tender and pork is fully cooked

Beef Bourguinon

Allergies: SF, GF, DF, EF

Ingredients -

- ❖ 3/4 or 1 pound cubed Lean Beef
- ❖ 1/4 cup red wine
- ❖ 2 Tbsp. coconut oil
- ❖ 1/4 tsp. thyme
- ❖ 1/4 tsp. black pepper
- ❖ 1 cloves garlic, crushed
- ❖ 1/2 onion, diced
- ❖ 1/3 pound mushrooms, sliced
- ❖ 2 Tbsp. cup almond flour

Instructions

- Marinate Beef in wine, oil, thyme, and pepper for a few hours at room temperature or 6-8 hours in the fridge.
- Cook garlic and onion in a pan until soft.
- Add mushrooms.
- Cook until they are browned.
- Drain beef liquid.
- Place Beef in the slow cooker.
- Sprinkle flour over the beef and stir to coat.
- Add the mushroom mixture on top.
- Pour reserved marinade over all. Cook on low for 7-9 hrs.

Italian Chicken

Allergies: SF, GF, DF, EF

Ingredients -

- ❖ 2 pieces of skinless ChickenChicken
- ❖ 2 Tbsp. almond flour

- 1/2 tsp. salt
- 1/8 tsp. pepper
- 1/4 cup chicken broth
- 1/2 cup sliced mushrooms
- 1/4 tsp. paprika
- 1/2 zucchini, sliced into medium pieces
- ground black pepper
- parsley to garnish

Instructions

- Season chicken with 1 tsp. Salt.
- Combine flour, pepper, remaining salt, and paprika. Coat chicken pieces with this mixture.
- Place zucchini first in a crockpot.
- Pour broth over zucchini.
- Arrange ChickenChicken on top.
- Cover and cook on Low for 6 to 8 hours or until tender.
- Turn control to high, add mushrooms, cover, and cook on high for additional 10-15 minutes.
- Garnish with parsley and ground black pepper.

Slow Cook Jambalaya

Allergies: SF, GF, DF, EF, NF

Ingredients -

- 1/2 Bell pepper, chopped
- 1/2 Onion, chopped
- 1 Medium tomato, chopped
- 1/2 cup Chopped celery
- 1 Clove garlic, crushed

- ❖ 1 tbsp. minced parsley
- ❖ 1 tbsp. Chopped thyme leaves
- ❖ 1 tbsp. chopped oregano leaves
- ❖ 1/8 tsp. Cayenne & 1/4 tsp. Salt
- ❖ 4 ounces pork, chopped
- ❖ 4 ounces Chicken breast, chopped
- ❖ 1 cups Beef broth
- ❖ 1/4 pound Cooked shelled shrimp
- ❖ 1/4 cup Cooked brown rice

Instructions

- Shell shrimp and halve lengthwise.
- Combine all ingredients except shrimp & rice in a slow cooker.
- Cover & cook on low 9-10 hours.
- Turn slow cooker on high, add cooked shrimp & cooked rice.
- Cover; cook on high 20-30 minutes.

Ropa Vieja

Allergies: SF, GF, DF, EF, NF

Ingredients -

- ❖ 1 tbsp. coconut oil
- ❖ 3/4 or 1 pound beef flank steak
- ❖ 1/2 cup beef broth
- ❖ 1/2 cup tomato sauce
- ❖ 1 small onion, sliced
- ❖ 1/2 green bell pepper sliced into strips
- ❖ 1 cloves garlic, chopped
- ❖ 1/4 cup tomato paste
- ❖ 1/2 tsp. ground cumin

❖ 1/2 tsp. chopped cilantro

❖ 1/2 tbsp. Olive oil or avocado oil & 1 tbsp. lemon juice

Instructions

● Heat oil in a skillet over high heat. Brown the flank steak on each side (4 minutes per side).

● Move the Beef to a slow cooker.

● Add in the beef broth and tomato sauce, then add the onion, bell pepper, garlic, tomato paste, cumin, cilantro, olive oil, and lemon juice.

● Stir until blended.

● Cover, and cook on high for 4 hours or on Low for up to 8 hours.

● When ready to serve, shred meat and serve with salad.

Lemon Roast Chicken

Allergies: SF, GF, DF, EF, NF

Ingredients -

❖ 2 pieces skinless ChickenChicken

❖ 1 dash Salt

❖ 1 dash Pepper

❖ 1 tsp. Oregano

❖ 1 cloves minced garlic

❖ 1 tbsp. coconut oil

❖ 1/4 cup water

❖ 1 tbsp. Lemon juice

❖ Rosemary

Instructions

● Wash Chicken and season with salt and pepper.

● Sprinkle half of oregano and garlic inside the chicken cavity.

- Add coconut oil to a frying pan.

- Brown Chicken on all sides and transfer to crockpot.

- Sprinkle with oregano and garlic.

- Add water to the frying pan and stir to loosen brown bits.

- Pour into the crockpot and cover.

- Cook on low 7 hours.

- Add lemon juice when cooking is done.

- Transfer chicken to cutting board and carve ChickenChicken.

- Skim fat. Pour the juice into the sauce bowl.

- Serve with rosemary and some juice over ChickenChicken.

Fall Lamb and Vegetable Stew

Allergies: SF, GF, DF, EF, NF

Ingredients -

- 3/4 or 1 pound Lamb stew meat
- 1 chopped Tomatoes
- 1/2 Summer squash
- 1/2 Zucchini
- 1/2 cup Mushrooms, sliced
- 1/2 cup Bell peppers, chopped
- 1/2 cup Onions, chopped
- 1/2 teaspoons Salt
- 1 Garlic cloves, crushed
- 1/4 tsp. Thyme leaves
- 1 Bay leaves
- 1 cups chicken broth

Instructions

- Cut squash and zucchini.

- Place vegetables and lamb in the crockpot.
- Mix salt, garlic, thyme, and bay leaf into the broth and pour over lamb and vegetables.
- Cover and cook on Low for 7 hours.

FISH

Cioppino

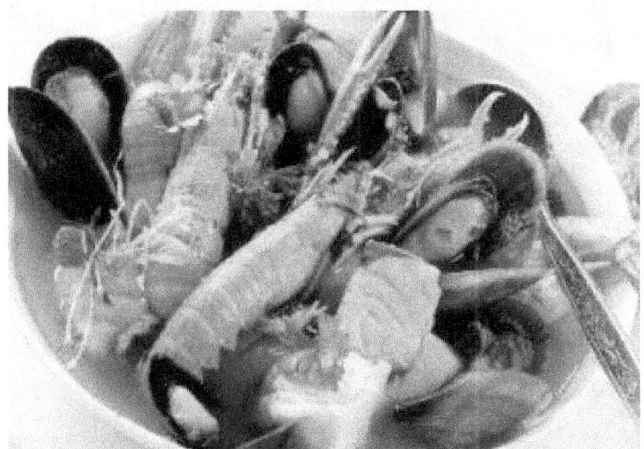

Allergies: SF, GF, DF, EF, NF

Ingredients -

- ❖ 1/4 cup coconut oil
- ❖ 1 onions, chopped
- ❖ 1 cloves garlic, minced
- ❖ 1/2 bunch fresh parsley, chopped
- ❖ 1/2 cup stewed tomatoes
- ❖ 1/2 cups chicken broth
- ❖ 1 bay leaves
- ❖ 1/2 tbsp. dried basil
- ❖ 1/4 tsp. dried thyme
- ❖ 1/4 tsp. dried oregano
- ❖ 1/2 cup water
- ❖ 1/2 cup white wine
- ❖ 1/2 pound peeled and deveined large shrimp
- ❖ 1/2 pound bay scallops
- ❖ 6 small clams
- ❖ 6 cleaned and debearded mussels
- ❖ 1/2 cups crabmeat

❖ 1/2 pounds cod fillets, cubed

Instructions

- Over medium heat, melt coconut oil in a large stockpot and add onions, parsley, and garlic. Cook slowly, stirring occasionally until onions are soft.
- Add tomatoes to the pot.
- Add chicken broth, oregano, bay leaves, basil, thyme, water, and wine.
- Mix well. Cover and simmer 30 minutes.
- Stir in the shrimp, scallops, clams, mussels, and crabmeat.
- Stir in fish.
- Bring to boil. Lower heat, cover and simmer until clams open.

Flounder with Orange Coconut Oil

Allergies: SF, GF, DF, EF, NF

Ingredients -

- ❖ 1 pound flounder
- ❖ 1 tbsp. white wine
- ❖ 1 tbsp. lemon juice
- ❖ 1 tbsp. coconut oil
- ❖ 1 tbsp. parsley
- ❖ 1/3 tsp. black pepper
- ❖ 1 tbsp. orange zest
- ❖ 1/4 tsp. salt
- ❖ 1/4 cup chopped scallions

Instructions

- Preheat oven to 325F. Sprinkle fish with pepper and salt.
- Place fish in the baking dish. Sprinkle orange zest on top of the fish.

- Melt remaining coconut oil and add the parsley and scallions to the coconut oil and pour over flounder.
- Then add in the white wine.
- Place in oven and bake for 15 minutes.
- Serve fish with extra juice on a side.

Grilled Salmon

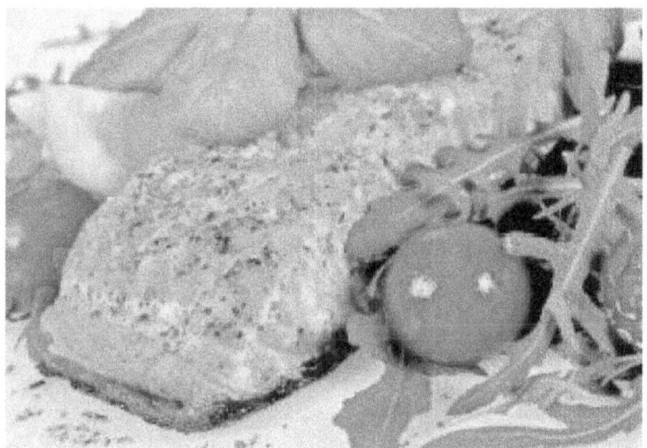

Allergies: SF, GF, DF, EF, NF

Ingredients -

- ❖ 2 salmon filets
- ❖ 2 Tbsp. coconut oil
- ❖ 1 tbsp. fish sauce
- ❖ 1 tbsp. lemon juice
- ❖ 1 tbsp. thinly sliced green onion
- ❖ 1 clove garlic, minced & 1/4 tsp. ground ginger
- ❖ 1/4 tsp. crushed red pepper flakes
- ❖ 1/4 tsp. sesame oil
- ❖ 1/8 tsp. Salt

Instructions

- Whisk together coconut oil, fish sauce, garlic, ginger, red chili flakes, lemon juice, green onions, sesame oil, and salt.
- Put fish in a glass dish, and pour marinade over.
- Cover and refrigerate for 4 hours.
- Preheat grill. Place salmon on the grill.
- Grill until fish becomes tender.
- Turn halfway during cooking.

Crab Cakes

Allergies: SF, GF, DF, NF

Ingredients -

- 1 lbs. crabmeat
- 1 beaten eggs
- 1 cup flax seeds meal
- 1 tbsp. mustard
- 1 tbsp. grated horseradish
- 1/4 cup coconut oil
- 1/2 tsp. lemon rind
- 1 tbsp. lemon juice
- 1 tbsp. parsley
- 1/4 tsp. cayenne pepper
- 1 tsp. fish sauce

Instructions

- In a medium bowl, combine all ingredients except oil.
- Shape into small hamburgers.
- In fry pan, heat oil and cook patties for 3-4 minutes on each side or until golden brown.
- Optionally, bake them in the oven.
- Serve as appetizers or as the main course with a large fiber salad.

SWEETS

Fruits dipped in chocolate.

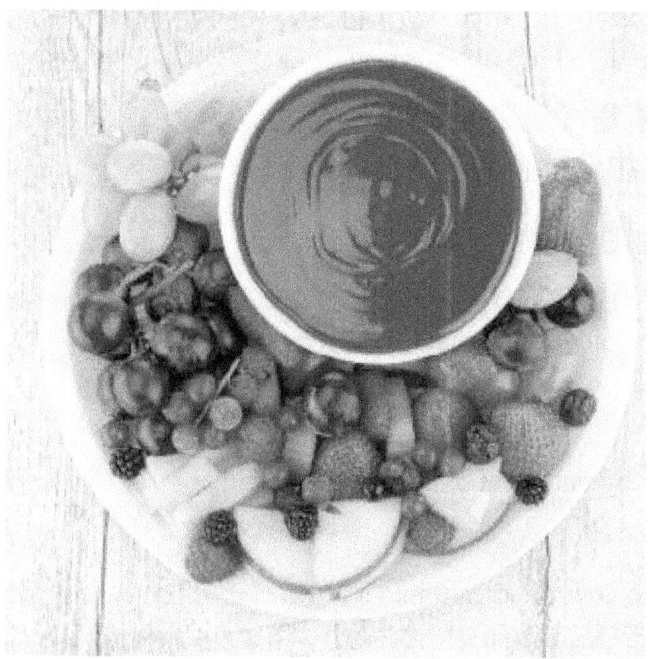

Allergies: SF, GF, DF, EF, V

Ingredients -

- ❖ 1 apple or 1 banana or a bowl of strawberries or any fruit that can be dipped in melted chocolate
- ❖ 1/2 cup of melted superfoods chocolate (see earlier recipe)
- ❖ 2 tbsp. chopped nuts (almond, walnut, Brazil nuts) or seeds (hemp, chia, sesame, flax meal)

Instructions

- Cut the apple in wedges or cut the banana in quarters.
- Melt the chocolate and chop the nuts.
- Dip fruit in chocolate, sprinkle with nuts or seeds, and lay on the tray.
- Transfer the tray to the fridge so the chocolate can harden; serve. If you don't want chocolate, cover fruits with almond or sunflower butter and sprinkle with chia or hemp seeds and cut it into chunks and serve.

Whipped Coconut cream

Allergies: SF, GF, DF, EF, V, NF

Ingredients -

- ❖ 2 cups of any fresh berries
- ❖ 1/2 lemons
- ❖ 1 can full-fat coconut milk (14 oz.), refrigerated overnight
- ❖ 1 tsp of ground vanilla bean
- ❖ 2 Tbsp. lucuma powder
- ❖ Dash of cardamom, nutmeg, and clove (optional)

Instructions

- Different coconut cream from the milk by putting it overnight in the fridge.
- Don't shake it before opening.
- Open the can of coconut milk and scrape out the cream into a bowl.
- Use the saved milk for smoothies or other recipes.
- Add cardamom, lucuma powder, and vanilla.
- Whip the cream with a hand mixer until fluffy. Put in the fridge.
- Wash berries and place them in serving bowls or glasses.
- Squeeze the lemon over the berries.
- Place a big scoop of cream on top of the berries and serve.

Ice cream

Allergies: SF, GF, DF, EF, V, NF

Freeze a banana cut into chunks and process it in a blender once frozen and add half a tsp. of cinnamon or 1 tsp. Of cocoa or both and eat it like ice-cream.

Other option would be to add one spoon of almond butter and mix it with mashed banana, it's also a delicious ice cream

CONCLUSION

If you have diabetes, your body cannot make or properly use insulin. This leads to high blood glucose, or blood sugar, levels. Healthy eating helps keep your blood sugar in your target range. It is a critical part of managing your diabetes because controlling your blood sugar can prevent the complications of diabetes.

A registered dietitian can help make an eating plan just for you. It should take into account your weight, medicines, lifestyle, and other health problems you have.

Healthy diabetic eating includes

- Limiting foods that are high in sugar
- Eating smaller portions, spread out over the day.
- Being careful about when and how many carbohydrates you eat
- Eating a variety of whole-grain foods, fruits, and vegetables every day.
- Eating less fat
- Limiting your use of alcohol
- Using less salt